THE
CARDIOLOGY ROTATION

THE
CARDIOLOGY
ROTATION

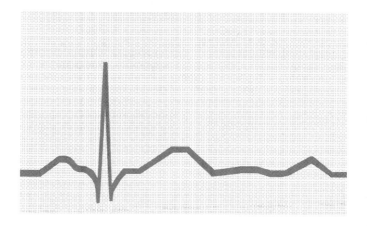

George J. Taylor, MD
Professor of Medicine
Medical University of South Carolina
Charleston, South Carolina

**Blackwell
Science**

Blackwell Science

©2001 by George J. Taylor

Editorial Offices:
Commerce Place, 350 Main Street, Malden,
Massachusetts 02148, USA
Osney Mead, Oxford OX2 0EL, England
25 John Street, London WC1N 2BL, England
23 Ainslie Place, Edinburgh EH3 6AJ, Scotland
54 University Street, Carlton, Victoria 3053, Australia

Other Editorial Offices:
Blackwell Wissenschafts-Verlag GmbH, Kurfürstendamm 57, 10707 Berlin, Germany
Blackwell Science KK, MG Kodenmacho Building, 7-10 Kodenmacho
Nihombashi, Chuo-ku, Tokyo 104, Japan
Iowa State University Press, A Blackwell Science Company, 2121 S. State Avenue, Ames,
Iowa 50014-8300, USA

Distributors:

USA
Blackwell Science, Inc.
Commerce Place
350 Main Street
Malden, Massachusetts 02148
(Telephone orders: 800-215-1000
or 781-388-8250;
fax orders: 781-388-8270)

Canada
Login Brothers Book Company
324 Saulteaux Crescent
Winnipeg, Manitoba R3J 3T2
(Telephone orders: 204-837-2987)

Australia
Blackwell Science Pty, Ltd.
54 University Street
Carlton, Victoria 3053
(Telephone orders: 03-9347-0300;
fax orders: 03-9349-3016)

Outside North America and Australia
Blackwell Science, Ltd.
c/o Marston Book Services, Ltd.
P.O. Box 269
Abingdon
Oxon OX14 4YN
England
(Telephone orders: 44-01235-465500;
fax orders: 44-01235-465555)

Acquisitions: Beverly Copland
Development: William Deluise
Production: Irene Herlihy
Manufacturing: Lisa Flanagan
Marketing Manager: Toni Fournier
Cover design by Hannus Design
Typeset by Gallagher
Printed and bound by DS Graphics

Printed in the United States of America
00 01 02 03 5 4 3 2 1

Library of Congress Cataloging-in-Publication Data
Taylor, George Jesse.
The cardiology rotation / by George J. Taylor.
    p. ;   cm
Includes index.
ISBN 0-632-04352-0
1. Heart—Pathophysiology. 2. Heart—Diseases—Diagnosis. I. Title.
[DNLM: 1. Cardiovascular Diseases. WG 120 T241c 2001]
RD682.9 .T39 2001
616.1′2—dc21   00-068002

For Marilyn, my best teacher

Contents

Preface

The Cardiology Rotation is for house officers and medical students who are doing an elective rotation on the cardiology service. It reviews the pathophysiology, physical diagnosis, and natural history of common cardiac ailments and provides an approach to diagnosis and treatment.

This book emphasizes fundamental issues, things that may not be explained clearly or in an organized fashion on a busy clinical service. For example, What is afterload? What is the difference between treating diastolic and systolic heart failure? How do I remember the many confusing facts about valvular disease? What does replacing the mitral valve do to cardiac loading and performance? What is the thallium scan and how does pharmacologic stress testing work? How do I advise my uncle about his cholesterol, and how does simvistatin lower LDL? What do they do in the electrophysiology lab (and does it have anything to do with EP doctors' eccentricity)? How should I evaluate the jugular venous pulse, the apical impulse, or the aortic second sound? How do you measure pulsus paradoxus?

The Cardiology Rotation is not a comprehensive review of heart disease. From my perspective working on the consult service for more than 20 years, I have selected illnesses that I know you will encounter, and concepts you should *understand* after your one-month rotation. It is also what you will likely find on board exams, and inclusion of new therapies and clinical trials make it a useful board review.

I am convinced that you will remember little about heart disease—and understand less—without knowledge of how the heart and circulation work. Plus, physiology is great sport. This book emphasizes basic mechanisms, but limits this to what is relevant to practice. (Sure, cellular electrophysiology is interesting, but you won't encounter it on the wards, so I do not discuss it.) I see patients and teach every day; trust me to choose and review the basic science that is clinically useful.

I suggest that you read through this book during your first week on the service. It is a fast way get the big picture, and to prepare for interaction with your learned colleague, the attending. As you see patients, you will refer back to specific sections and will flesh out your understanding by reading review articles (the bulk of the references). Use the library, and do not buy encyclopedic cardiology texts early in your career; they are too long, too heavy, too expensive, and out of date in a couple of years.

A one-month cardiology rotation is your opportunity to learn to read electrocardiograms (ECGs). Ideally, there will be a formal ECG reading experience with an attending. If not, consider the text *150 Practice ECGs* (Blackwell Science, 1997), which provides an introductory manual plus enough practice tracings to help you become proficient. There is little overlap with this book, and the two together constitute a basic curriculum for the cardiology rotation.

GJT
Charleston, SC
November, 2000

CHAPTER 1

Congestive Heart Failure

CONGESTIVE HEART FAILURE CAUSED BY SYSTOLIC DYSFUNCTION _____

Epidemiology and Natural History

Congestive heart failure (CHF) is the clinical syndrome caused by insufficient cardiac output, leading to either pulmonary or systemic congestion. Extracardiac or valvular heart disease may limit cardiac output, even though ventricular function is normal. Rare cases of CHF with high cardiac output occur (Table 1.1). This chapter is about CHF caused by ventricular dysfunction. Isolated failure of the right ventricle (RV) causes peripheral edema and splanchnic congestion. Left ventricular (LV) failure causes pulmonary congestion, including exertional dyspnea, orthopnea, paroxysmal nocturnal dyspnea, and eventually pulmonary edema. Easy fatigue and exercise intolerance are early and often subtle manifestations of both left and right heart failure.

About 400,000 new cases of CHF are diagnosed annually in the United States. It is the most common admitting diagnosis for elderly people, and the incidence of CHF more than doubles with each decade over age 45. This trend will progress because reduced mortality in middle age from coronary artery disease leaves an older population at risk.

Coronary artery disease is the most common cause of LV systolic dysfunction and CHF (Table 1.1). Hypertension used to be the most common cause, but more effective treatment of asymptomatic hypertension has changed this. An interesting and recently discovered cause of LV dysfunction is incessant supraventricular tachycardia (this is just now making it to board examinations and is a favorite clinical pearl on housestaff rounds). Typically, a patient with rapid atrial fibrillation lasting at least 3 to

TABLE 1.1. Causes of CHF

Illnesses that inhibit ventricular filling but do not affect ventricular function (result: low cardiac output)
- Mitral stenosis (blocks LV filling)
- Pericardial tamponade or constriction (blocks RV filling)

Conditions influencing ventricular function, altering either preload or afterload (result: low cardiac output)
- Aortic stenosis (high LV afterload)
- Aortic regurgitation (LV volume overload)
- Mitral regurgitation (LV volume overload)
- Pulmonic stenosis (high RV afterload)
- Tricuspid regurgitation (RV volume overload)
- Hypertensive heart disease (high LV afterload)
- Primary pulmonary hypertension (high RV afterload)
- Secondary pulmonary hypertension (high RV afterload caused by cor pulmonale, left heart failure, or the Eisenmenger's syndrome)

Illnesses primarily affecting LV systolic (contractile) dysfunction (result: low cardiac output)
- Coronary artery disease (myocardial infarction)
- Idiopathic dilated cardiomyopathy
- Tachycardia-induced cardiomyopathy (atrial fibrillation, incessant supraventricular tachycardia, or ventricular tachycardia)
- Viral myocarditis (coxsackie A and B, echovirus, influenza A and B, polio virus, arbovirus, cytomegalovirus, mumps)
- Acute rheumatic fever ("rheumatic myocarditis")
- Other bacterial and fungal infections
- Toxins (alcohol, cocaine, heroin, amphetamines, ethylene glycol, cobalt, lead, arsenic)
- Drugs (Adriamycin, cyclophosphamides, sulfonamides, ipecac)
- Nutritional deficiencies (protein, thiamine, selenium, L-carnitine)
- Electrolyte disorders (low sodium, calcium, magnesium, or phosphate)
- Collagen vascular disease (lupus, rheumatoid arthritis, periarteritis nodosa, Reiter's syndrome, systemic sclerosis, Takayasu's syndrome, hypersensitivity vasculitis)
- Endocrine disorders (diabetes, hypo/hyperthyroidism, pheochromo-cytoma, hypoparathyroidism)
- Miscellaneous (peripartum cardiomyopathy, sleep apnea, hypereosino-philic syndrome, giant cell myocarditis)

Illnesses causing LV diastolic dysfunction (result: inadequate LV filling and low cardiac output)
- Idiopathic diastolic dysfunction (usually elderly women)
- Hypertension
- Any cardiac condition that increases afterload and induces ventricular hypertrophy
- Hypertrophic cardiomyopathy (including idiopathic hypertrophic subaortic stenosis)
- Infiltrative cardiomyopathies or myocardial fibrosis (amyloidosis, sarcoidosis, hemochromatosis, other inflammatory conditions, including collagen vascular disease)

table continues

4 weeks has a low ejection fraction (EF) on the echocardiogram. After control of the ventricular rate there is gradual improvement in LVEF over the next month. Multiple other causes of LV dysfunction are surveyed in Table 1.1.

TABLE 1.1. *(continued)*

High-output heart failure (in most cases high cardiac output alone does not cause CHF but precipitates it when there is underlying heart disease)
Anemia
Thyrotoxicosis
Arteriovenous fistulas (after trauma, arteriovenous fistula for hemodialysis, Osler-Weber-Rendu disease, rupture of an aortic aneurysm into the inferior vena cava)
Beriberi (thiamine deficiency may contribute to alcoholic heart disease; consider thiamine treatment when the cause of heart failure is obscure or there is an unusual dietary history)
Paget's disease of bone

The natural history of CHF is somewhat difficult to define because of patient selection bias and changes in therapy. The Framingham Study, conducted between 1949 and 1971, included patients with both mild and severe CHF and showed a 40% 3-year mortality. This study was based on a clinical diagnosis, and few of the patients had documentation of LV function; it probably included patients who did not have CHF. In contrast, a trial conducted by a heart failure research group between 1979 and 1984 focused on patients with proven LV dysfunction and severe CHF and found a 75% 3-year mortality.

A sense of the natural history of CHF in the more modern era of angiotensin-converting enzyme (ACE) inhibitors is apparent from the placebo arms of randomized trials (Table 1.2), with mortality rates of about one third during 2 to 4 years of follow-up. These trials also found that the severity of symptoms parallels mortality, with class III and IV patients at highest risk (Table 1.2).

A reduction in CHF mortality in recent years can be attributed to ACE inhibitor therapy and the avoidance of type I antiarrhythmic agents (note CAST trial in Chapter 5). Beta blockade, attention to electrolytes, and more effective treatment of ventricular arrhythmias also reduce mortality.

Pathophysiology
Ventricular Anatomy and Function
The left ventricle is thicker than the right ventricle. It works against a much higher pressure load, or "afterload." You know that weight lifting builds muscle mass. What is true for the weight-lifter's arms is true for heart muscle as well. Because aortic pressure is much higher than pulmonary artery pressure, the left

TABLE 1.2. Effect of Afterload Reduction Therapy on Survival in CHF

Trial	n	Inclusion Criteria*	Therapy	Mean Follow-up (mo)	Treatment Mortality	Placebo Mortality
VHeFT-I	642	NYHA II-III EF < 45%, CTR > 0.55	hydralazine/isordil vs. prazosin vs. placebo	30	25% (hydralazine/isordil)	34%
CONSENSUS	253	NYHA IV	Enalapril vs. placebo	6	25%	44%
VHeFT-II	804	NYHA II-III	Hydralazine/isordil vs. enalapril	24	18% enalapril, 25% hydralazine/isordil	NA
SOLVED	2561	NYHA II-III EF < 35%	Enalapril vs. placebo	42	35.2%	39.7%

*The New York Heart Association (NYHA) functional classification: I, no symptoms with physical activity but known disease; II, slight limitation of activity, and symptoms with physical activity; III, symptoms with minimal activity and marked limitation of activity; IV, symptoms at rest, and symptoms with any physical activity.

TABLE 1.3. Determinants of Cardiac Output and Stroke Volume

Cardiac output (mL/min) = Heart rate (beats/min) × Stroke volume (mL/beat)
Stroke volume is augmented (+) or depressed (−) by three factors:

1. (+) Preload = the ventricular load or volume at the end of diastole. (Higher preload augments stroke volume.)
2. (−) Afterload = the load or resistance against which the ventricle empties during systole. (Higher afterload impedes the ventricle's ability to empty, lowering stroke volume.)
3. (+) Contractility = the basic state of ventricular muscle (its innate ability to contract independent of loading conditions—increased contractility means greater ventricular emptying and greater stroke volume).

4

ventricle is more muscular than the right. Raising afterload increases the muscle mass of either of the ventricles, and lowering it allows a reduction in muscle mass.

The labels "right" and "left" ventricle do not accurately describe the position of the heart in the chest. Actually, the right ventricle is in front of (anterior to) the left ventricle, and the plane of the interventricular septum is roughly parallel to the chest wall, positions that are apparent from the echocardiogram. The right ventricular (RV) impulse, when palpable, is felt along the left parasternal border, and the right ventricle is the first chamber punctured with an intracardiac injection.

Normally, the interventricular septum acts as a part of the left ventricle. When you think about it, the septum has to "choose sides," because it is anatomically a part of both ventricles. It chooses the side that is working hardest, normally the left ventricle. On the echo (or with other imaging studies that show the heart in motion), the septum moves toward the posterior wall of the left ventricle during systole and away from the free wall of the right ventricle. Conditions that produce RV overload or failure may lead to a reversal of this normal pattern, with the septum moving toward the right ventricle and away from the left ventricle during systole (this "paradoxical septal motion" is common with the volume overload of atrial septal defect, for example).

Cardiac Output and Ventricular Function

When all is said and done, what the body wants from the pump is blood flow. Output is the product of heart rate and the "stroke volume," the volume ejected with each heartbeat. The units of measurement are fairly simple (Table 1.3). Increasing heart rate is an important early compensatory mechanism, the normal response to reduced cardiac output. In a normal young person cardiac output goes up with increasing heart rate until the rate reaches 170 to 180 beats/min and then it falls off (because there is not enough time between beats for ventricular filling). An elderly person with cardiac dysfunction may have cardiac output fall at rates above 150 beats/min. When I see a patient with CHF and resting tachycardia, a rate above 100 beats/min, I know that LV function is depressed, and prognosis poor.

Three things influence ventricular stroke volume: preload, afterload, and contractility.

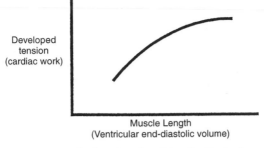

FIGURE 1.1. Ventricular function describing Starling's observation relating preload (muscle fiber length or ventricular volume just *before* ventricular contraction) and stroke volume (one measure of cardiac work) when the ventricle is then stimulated. With increased muscle fiber length, the strength of contraction increases.

Preload Precisely defined, preload is the length of each muscle fiber *before* contraction. When a strip of muscle is stimulated, it twitches and generates tension that can be measured. Within physiologic limits (meaning that the muscle is not overstretched to the point of injury), increasing the resting length produces a stronger contraction (Fig. 1.1). A century ago, Starling and others showed that this is as true for heart muscle as for skeletal muscle.

In the intact heart, muscle fiber length is proportional to ventricular diastolic volume. Thus, increased ventricular filling during diastole is the same as increased preload and leads to more forceful contraction when the ventricle is stimulated. That is why volume expansion (salt and water retention) is a basic compensatory mechanism in heart failure. Increased vascular volume means increased venous return to both ventricles, an increase in ventricular diastolic volume, and higher stroke volume.

Because increasing preload increases stroke volume and cardiac output, it would seem that treatments to expand volume would be useful when ventricular function is depressed. The problem with this is that there is a limit to how much volume can be tolerated. When salt and water are retained and the pulmonary capillary hydrostatic pressure exceeds 25 mm Hg, the oncotic pressure that keeps fluid in the vascular space is overcome, and fluid is pushed into the interstitial space. Pulmonary congestion thus places a limit on the Starling mechanism's capacity to compensate for low cardiac output.

When considering ventricular "function," it is natural to think primarily of the contractile process. There often is confusion about "diastolic function" and "ventricular compliance." These terms relate to how easily the ventricle fills during diastole, when it is relaxed, and have nothing to do with ventricular contraction. But diastolic properties are closely related to preload and stroke volume (Fig. 1.2). A compliant ventricle fills easily, allowing adequate preloading of the ventricle (stretching of muscle fibers) to generate stroke volume. A stiff ("noncompliant") ventricle may not accommodate an adequate blood volume, and stroke volume suffers. Abnormal stiffness, or diastolic dysfunction, may result from hypertrophy, infiltrative cardiomyopathy, or ischemia.

Think about the contribution of the "atrial kick." Contraction of the atria at the end of diastole provides the last increment of ventricular filling, increasing preload and stroke volume (Fig. 1.3). When atrial contraction is lost, as with atrial fibrillation or ventricular pacing, preload, stroke volume, and cardiac output fall. For a person with normal diastolic function, loss of atrial contraction causes a 10% to 15% drop in cardiac output.

On the other hand, a patient with *diastolic dysfunction* relies more on atrial contraction to fill the ventricle. A stiff ventricle resists passive filling during diastole, and atrial contraction provides a larger than normal proportion of filling. In such cases, a loss of the atrial kick may cause cardiac output to fall more than 25%. *Patients with stiff ventricles are said to be "preload dependent" and are especially susceptible to volume depletion or loss of atrial contraction.* This explains why a patient with aortic valve stenosis and LV hypertrophy (LVH) may experience a fall in blood pressure with the development of atrial fibrillation.

Afterload This is the load the ventricle works against when it contracts, during systole. Aortic or pulmonic valve stenosis impede flow and raise afterload, and both induce ventricular hypertrophy. In the absence of ventricular outflow tract obstruction, vascular resistance and blood pressure provide rough approximations of afterload. Patients with hypertension have increased afterload, and LV hypertrophy is the basis of hypertensive heart disease.

On the other hand, afterload may be reduced with no apparent change in blood pressure. Ohm's law states that *pressure = flow × resistance*. Thus, a vasodilator drug that lowers resistance by

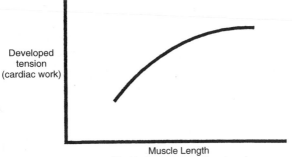

A. Basis for Starlings' Law of the Heart

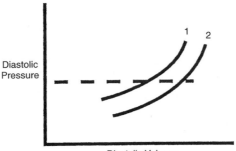

B. Influence of ventricular compliance on diastolic volume

FIGURE 1.2. (A) A restatement of Starling's law: Increased resting muscle length *before* stimulation leads to increased strength of contraction and developed tension once the muscle is stimulated. In the intact heart, ventricular volume may be substituted for muscle fiber length, and any measure of cardiac work may be substituted for developed tension. (Rough measures of cardiac work would include ventricular stroke volume, cardiac output, and ejection fraction.) (B) Compliance of the ventricle during diastole influences ventricular filling. At a given ventricular diastolic pressure, patient 1 has a lower ventricular volume (and therefore muscle fiber length) than patient 2. Patient 1 has a stiffer, less compliant ventricle.

figure continues

20% but allows cardiac output (flow) to increase by 20% causes no change in blood pressure. That is why vasodilator therapy may be used in patients with advanced CHF and low blood pressure.

On the ventricular function curve, a reduction in afterload produces a shift up and to the left (Fig. 1.4). Reducing afterload

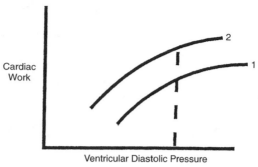

C. Ventricular function curve, substituting diastolic pressure for volume

FIGURE 1.2. (*continued*) (C) In practice, it is easier to measure ventricular diastolic pressure than volume. Because the two are roughly proportional, pressure is substituted for volume on the ventricular function curve. But altered diastolic compliance may cause an apparent shift in the curve. Patient 1 appears to have worse ventricular function than patient 2, and that would be the case if diastolic compliance is the same for both. But if patient 1 has a stiffer ventricle (as in B), end-diastolic volume may be lower than it is for patient 2. In this case, at equal ventricular volumes, the two might have identical systolic function and therefore identical ventricular function curves. This illustrates the potential problem of substituting diastolic pressure for diastolic volume on the abscissa of the LV function curve.

with vasodilator therapy improves ventricular performance and cardiac output without increasing the myocardium's workload.

Hypertrophy, Wall Tension, and Myocardial Oxygen Demand The heart responds to increased afterload with an increase in contractility and, eventually, with hypertrophy. Myocardial oxygen demand is proportional to wall tension, and tension is determined by the interplay of ventricular pressure and size described by Laplace's law (Table 1.4). A dilated ventricle thus has higher wall tension than a smaller one and requires more oxygen. (A dilated aorta, loop of bowel, pulmonary bleb, or uterus all have increased wall tension and are thus more prone to rupture; Laplace's law applies to many areas of medicine.)

Contractility This third determinant of stroke volume is defined as an increase in the force of contraction when both preload and afterload are constant. Another name for contractility is the "inotropic" state. At the cellular level, calcium ions interact with the contractile proteins. When excitation leads to increased

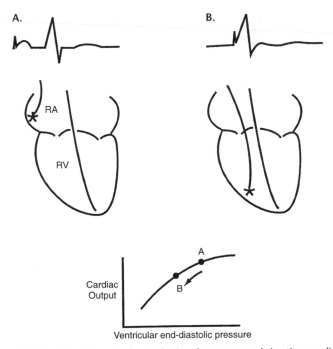

FIGURE 1.3. This simple study is often repeated in the cardiac catheterization laboratory. The heart is paced at a rate just above its baseline, and cardiac output is measured. (A) When the pacemaker is in the right atrium, atrial contraction is preserved (a P wave follows the pacer spike). (B) Pacing from the right ventricle leads to a loss of the P wave and atrial contraction. Ventricular diastolic pressure and volume decline—with this drop in preload—and cardiac output falls. On the LV function curve, the patient shifts from point A to point B (bottom).

calcium influx, contractility is augmented (as with digitalis or catecholamines); reduced calcium influx depresses contractility (as with the calcium channel blocker, verapamil, and β-adrenergic blockers).

On the ventricular function curve, an increase in contractility leads to a shift in the curve to the left. There is an increase in stroke volume for a given preload (Fig. 1.4).

Ejection Fraction (EF) A common measure of systolic function is ejection fraction, or that portion of blood ejected from the ventricle during systole. Thus, if the left ventricle contains 150 mL at the end of diastole and 50 mL at the end of systole, the LVEF is 67% and the stroke volume is 100 mL. It may be calculated by measuring the volume of the left ventricle at end-diastole

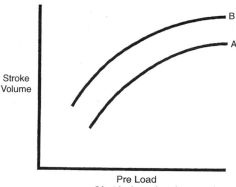

Stroke Volume

Pre Load
(Ventricular volume)

FIGURE 1.4. Manipulations that alter the ventricular function curve. Increasing *contractility* or reducing *afterload* shift the curve up and to the left, from curve A to curve B. Thus, with either manipulation stroke volume is higher for a given preload. For this reason, drugs that augment contractility or reduce afterload are useful therapies for CHF. What about diuretics? They reduce vascular volume and thus reduce preload; the ventricular function curve does not shift, and the patient moves down and to the left on the same curve. Stroke volume falls, but this is a necessary intervention to reduce pulmonary congestion.

TABLE 1.4. **Chamber Size, Wall Tension, and Pressure: Laplace's Law (A Physical Principle that Applies to Many Areas of Medicine)**

The law of Laplace describes the determinants of wall stress ("tension") and applies to any "container" of a fluid volume that has measurable intracavitary pressure. This would include chambers of the heart, blood vessels, airways, loops of bowel, the uterus, etc.

Wall stress = (Pressure) (Radius) / 2 (Wall thickness)

When applied to the left ventricle, wall stress (tension) is proportional to myocardial oxygen demand (MVO_2). A dilated left ventricle or one with pressure overload requires more oxygen. Increased LV thickness, hypertrophy, tends to "normalize" wall stress, and therefore MVO_2, of the pressure overloaded or dilated left ventricle.

This relationship is also important when gauging the possibility of rupture of an aneurysm, dilated loop of bowel, pulmonary bleb, etc. The higher the wall stress, the greater the chance of rupture. The size of the chamber (radius) determines the "burst" pressure. Increased wall thickness reduces the chance of rupture. Thus, a thin-walled LV aneurysm is more likely to rupture than an equally dilated left ventricle with normal wall thickness.

and again at end-systole using either the LV angiogram or echocardiogram. It may also be measured with radionuclide techniques, measuring radioisotope counts at end-diastole and end-systole and doing the arithmetic (see Box 1.1).

EF is a measure of muscle shortening, and like stroke volume, it depends on both contractility and loading conditions. Increased contractility and reduced afterload both increase EF. However, stroke volume and EF cannot be equated. A dilated left ventricle with a diastolic volume of 210 mL and an EF of 33% has a stroke volume of 70 mL. So does a normal ventricle of 140 mL and an EF of 50%. This simple math indicates another way that ventricular dilatation compensates for LV dysfunction.

Neurohormonal Response to Low Cardiac Output

CHF due to systolic dysfunction is instigated by some insult to LV pump function, but it is the complex interplay of neuroendocrine compensatory mechanisms that determine the severity of

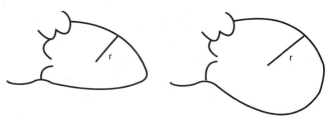

FIGURE 1.5. Ventricular remodeling. The left ventricle is normally an ellipsoid (left). With the development of cardiomyopathy it enlarges and also changes shape, becoming more spherical (right). Both changes increase the radius of curvature (r), and this increases wall tension (see Table 1.4 for a description of Laplace's law). Wall tension is proportional to myocardial oxygen demand, so the remodeling process aggravates LV dysfunction.

symptoms. Best understood are the adrenergic nervous system and the renin-angiotensin-aldosterone system. They are known to cross-regulate, with activation of one leading to activation of the other.

The immediate goal is maintenance of cardiac output and flow to vital organs (primarily the kidneys). Increased sympathetic tone increases heart rate and contractility. Decreased renal blood flow turns on the renin-angiotensin-aldosterone system. Aldosterone promotes salt and water retention, thus boosting intravascular volume, ventricular preload, and LV stroke volume. Activation of both the adrenergic and renin-angiotensin systems causes vasoconstriction that helps to maintain blood pressure and flow.

These responses to depressed flow help restore cardiac output over the short term. However, over the long run there may be adverse consequences: Increased peripheral resistance, and, hence, increased afterload, further depresses systolic performance. The eccentric hypertrophy and dilatation that occur as a result of stimulation by both of these neuroendocrine systems contribute to *ventricular remodeling*, a change in the shape of the ventricle that increases wall tension and therefore myocardial oxygen demand via the Laplace mechanism (Fig. 1.5). Increases in ventricular size and contractility raise the metabolic demands of the muscle. There also appears to be direct myocellular toxicity, possibly mediated by β-adrenergic mechanisms, which leads to myocardial cell death and eventual fibrosis. Additionally, myocytes may be lost secondary to "apoptosis," or programmed cell death, the result of excessive growth stimulation by cytokines that are expressed in some patients with CHF.

History and Physical Examination

Left heart failure causes progressively more severe pulmonary congestion: dyspnea with exertion, then orthopnea, then paroxysmal nocturnal dyspnea, then dyspnea at rest and pulmonary edema. Right heart failure causes peripheral and splanchnic congestion. You hear that LV failure is the most common cause of RV failure, and it is true. Curiously, an occasional patient with biventricular failure has severe peripheral edema and ascites with minimal or no pulmonary congestion. CHF in elderly patients may present as fatigue or a change in exercise tolerance, with little congestion.

History taking should include a survey for conditions that may cause or aggravate CHF: myocardial infarction with few or subtle symptoms, viral illnesses, a family history of cardiomyopathy, alcohol use, and gastrointestinal symptoms that would suggest blood loss and anemia.

General Examination

Note the overall state of health and vigor. Experienced clinicians know that frailty is not a nebulous physical finding, and its presence indicates a poor cardiac prognosis.

Cardiac cachexia is a diagnosis of exclusion. When weight loss develops in a patient with chronic heart failure, you must first exclude another etiology. Remember that occult bacterial endocarditis may cause weight loss in a patient with valvular disease. The pathophysiology of cachexia caused by heart failure is multifactorial. Anorexia is a common symptom of right heart failure because of splanchnic and hepatic congestion. Rarely, right heart failure may cause protein-losing enteropathy. Severe salt restriction may aggravate anorexia, because food does not taste as good. Digitalis toxicity may contribute to anorexia, and this can be a factor even when the digoxin level is in the therapeutic range. There may also be increased caloric needs. Both increased cardiac work (e.g., aortic stenosis or regurgitation) and the increased work of breathing with chronic pulmonary congestion raise caloric needs. More recently, patients with chronic heart failure have been found to have higher levels of the proinflammatory cytokine, *tumor necrosis factor,* and this may contribute to cachexia. Important physical findings include bitemporal and hypothenar wasting.

Vital Signs

Resting tachycardia is a powerful sign of decompensation in a patient with chronic CHF. Hypotension and narrow pulse pressure often accompany low stroke volume. Wide pulse pressure, on the other hand, is a finding of aortic regurgitation.

Jugular Venous Pulse

There are three parts to this examination: estimation of venous pressure, testing for abdominojugular reflux, and assessment of the venous waveform.

Venous Pressure The sternal angle, or angle of Lewis, is 5 cm above the level of the right atrium. Thus, if the top of the distended vein is 3 cm above the sternal angle, right atrial pressure is 8 cm H_2O. Pressure greater than 7 to 8 cm of water is abnormal. The patient may be examined in any position: With high pressure, you may not see the top of the venous column unless the patient is sitting upright. With low pressure, it may be necessary to have the patient almost flat to see a distended vein.

To be precise, the venous pressure that reflects RV filling pressure is not at the peak of the venous pulse wave but at about the midpoint of its total excursion. It thus excludes the bulk of the A wave, created by atrial contraction. In practice, this may be hard to gauge, and the small correction that it represents rarely makes the difference between a normal and an elevated pressure.

In most cases, high venous pressure indicates high right atrial pressure. An exception is *superior vena cava obstruction.* In this case, there is no venous pulsation, because the veins are isolated from the heart. Furthermore, the vein fills from above and not from below.

Abdominal-Jugular Test (AJT) Abdominojugular reflux is also called hepatojugular reflux. The maneuver is performed with the patient breathing normally (and not holding the breath). Push down on the periumbilical area for 10 seconds. In normal subjects, the venous pressure rises less than 3 cm and only transiently. A greater and more sustained rise occurs with *both right and left heart failure* and with tricuspid regurgitation. Although classically proposed as a test for *right heart* failure, one study found that patients with a positive AJT had elevation of both pulmonary wedge and right atrial pressures (probably because right heart failure is usually caused by left heart failure).

The AJT is especially useful in determining the cause of peripheral edema when there is no jugular venous distention. If the AJT is negative, heart failure is excluded. The edema must be from some other cause (e.g., calcium blocker therapy, veno-occlusive disease, low albumin, lymphatic obstruction).

Jugular Venous Pulse Waveform Recall that there is no valve separating the right atrium from the superior vena cava and jugular veins. Thus, atrial contraction pushes blood back to the veins as well as forward through the open tricuspid valve. Venous pressure waves are conveniently labeled: The A wave is generated by atrial contraction and the V wave, by ventricular contraction (Fig. 1.6).

To examine the pulse, have the patient breathe normally in a position where you can see venous pulsation through the sternocleidomastoid muscle (the internal jugular pulse) or pulsation of the more easily seen external jugular vein. Feel the brachial pulse while watching the vein to tell systole from diastole. *If the dominant venous pulse is before the brachial pulse (arterial systole), it is an A wave. If the dominant pulse is simultaneous with the arterial pulse, it is a V wave.* On the chart I state what I have observed: "JVP: A > V" (a normal exam) or "V > A" (an abnormal finding).

The V wave is created by ventricular systole, by either backward bulging of the tricuspid valve leaflets or slight backward movement of the valve ring during ventricular contraction. The wave is normally quite small. With an incompetent tricuspid valve the ventricle is no longer isolated from the atrium during systole, and ventricular systolic pressure is transmitted back to the neck veins (Fig. 1.6). A big V wave is not a subtle finding, and you have only to document that the dominant venous pulse wave is systolic (simultaneous with the arterial pulse). Look for a pulsatile liver and holosystolic murmur to confirm tricuspid regurgitation.

A giant A wave indicates high RV diastolic pressures. This usually occurs with pulmonary hypertension (the Eisenmenger syndrome, primary pulmonary hypertension, or recurrent pulmonary emboli) or with pulmonic valve stenosis. Tricuspid valve stenosis or atresia is a rare but potential cause. RV failure does not cause a giant A wave unless there is also pulmonary hypertension.

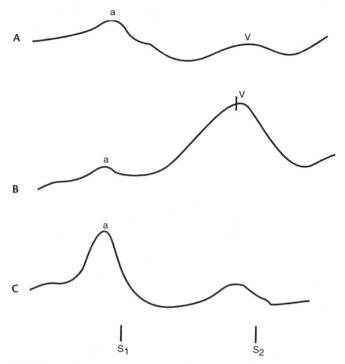

FIGURE 1.6. Jugular venous tracings from three patients. (A) Normal. The A wave is taller than the V wave. (B) Tricuspid regurgitation. There is a giant V wave, with transmission of RV pressure to the jugular veins because of the incompetent tricuspid valve. (C) Pulmonary hypertension. There is a giant A wave caused by elevated RV (and therefore right atrial) diastolic pressure.

Be aware that the A wave in a normal person may be of such low amplitude that it is not visible. Instead, the most obvious event may be the collapse of the venous column after atrial contraction, at a time of rapid filling of the now-empty atrium. This prominent x descent occurs early during ventricular systole and is a normal finding.

Examination of the Chest
Inspection of the chest and the pattern of breathing shows little abnormality when CHF is mild or moderate. *Cheyne-Stokes respiration,* a cyclical breathing pattern with progressively deeper breaths followed by a brief period of apnea, may occur with

advanced heart failure. It is caused, in part, by decreased sensitivity of the respiratory center of the brain to CO_2 and is more likely to develop in patients with cerebral pathology. It is aggravated by anything that further depresses the respiratory center, including sleep, narcotics, and some sedatives (particularly barbiturates).

Advanced obstructive lung disease with a barrel-shaped deformity of the chest may point to cor pulmonale as the cause of right heart failure. Kyphoscoliosis may also cause cor pulmonale.

Increased respiratory rate and greater effort of breathing may accompany severe pulmonary congestion and obstructive lung disease. *Patients with emphysema and hyperexpansion may not have audible rales with congestion; the chest x-ray is needed to exclude congestion.*

Pleural effusion may be a sign of either right heart or left heart congestion. The pleural space is drained by both the systemic and pulmonary circulations. Physical findings include deviation of the trachea away from the effusion, absence of fremitus (palpable breath sounds), dullness to percussion, and softer or absent breath sounds. Heart failure is the most common cause of effusion; when it is unilateral, it usually occurs on the right side. An isolated left-sided effusion suggests a noncardiac etiology.

Rales may be caused by heart or lung disease. I frequently hear inexperienced examiners describe rales as either "wet" (cardiac) or "dry" (pulmonary). However, when dealing with fine crackles, it is impossible to distinguish between the two based only on the quality of the sounds. More reliable is the *timing* of rales. With heart failure and early pulmonary congestion, fine crackles occur late in inspiration ("end-inspiratory rales"), and they are best heard at the bases of the lungs. Pulmonary fibrosis also causes fine crackles, but these rales are usually heard throughout inspiration ("pan-inspiratory rales"). The rales of pulmonary fibrosis may be isolated to the apices of the lungs or audible throughout the chest.

It helps to understand the mechanism of rales in heart failure with *interstitial* congestion. You are not hearing bubbles. Instead, the crackles are caused by the opening of collapsed airways. In the absence of congestion, there is little airway closure during expiration (Fig. 1.7). But lungs heavy with interstitial congestion have closure of small airways at a higher lung volume than is usual (it is the weight of the interstitium that is the problem). Thus, the airways close during normal expiration. To use the pulmonary

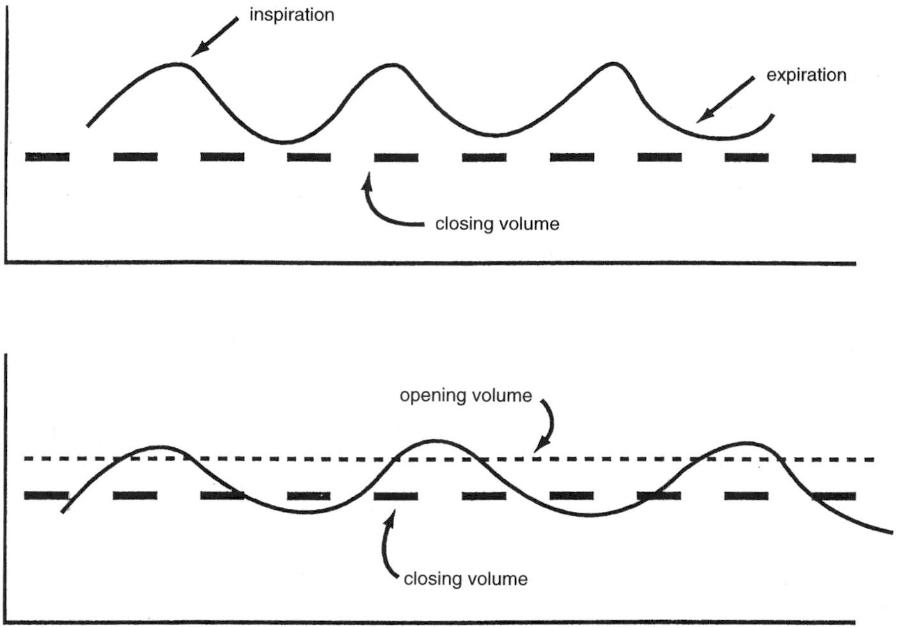

FIGURE 1.7. The pathophysiology of rales in congestive heart failure. In the normal state (top), the lung volume at which airways start to collapse, the "closing volume," is not reached during normal expiration. Pulmonary congestion changes this (bottom). The waterlogged lungs weigh heavily on the airways, and they collapse at a higher lung volume. Because the threshold for airway collapse has risen, the small airways close during normal expiration. Even greater volumes is needed to pop the collapsed airways open, and that happens nearer to the end of inspiration. For this reason, the inspiratory crackles of *interstitial* congestion occur at *end-inspiration*.

physiology term, there is elevated "closing volume." With subsequent inspiration, an even higher lung volume is needed to pop open the collapsed units, and the rales are thus end-inspiratory.

Wheezing is usually a sign of airway obstruction. It may develop in a patient with pulmonary congestion ("cardiac asthma"). Occasionally, an acutely ill older patient with wheezing and severe dyspnea may not have audible rales. The absence of a history of asthma points to the cardiac diagnosis, and the chest x-ray readily confirms pulmonary edema.

Abdomen and Extremities

Hepatomegaly and peripheral edema are signs of right heart failure. When it develops rapidly, the swollen liver may be tender. Ascites may develop with chronic congestion, especially when caused by constrictive pericarditis or tricuspid regurgitation. In such cases there may also be splenomegaly.

Pitting edema is found over the lower legs in the ambulatory patient. The bedridden patient may have peripheral edema only in the sacral area. When checking for edema I avoid hard pressure; gentle kneading with a finger tip effectively elicits pitting, and this approach seems more sophisticated than aggressively mashing the patient's swollen leg. Edema caused by heart failure is bilateral, and unilateral edema suggests venous obstruction.

Cardiac Examination
Apical Impulse

The location of the point of maximum impulse (PMI) should be determined with the patient lying flat. Its normal location is the midclavicular line and fifth intercostal space. It is tapping in quality and occupies a space of no more than 2 cm. LVH may not displace the PMI, but it becomes more forceful, like a fist hitting your hand. Systolic dysfunction and LV volume overload and dilatation cause displacement of the PMI toward the anterior axillary line and enlargement of the apex beat so that it may be felt in more than one interspace. The volume overload apical impulse is diffuse and rocking in quality.

An RV impulse is not palpable in normal patients. RV pressure or volume overload produces a "lift" along the left parasternal border. When the lift is forceful and sustained, it suggests pressure overload. Volume overload causes a lift that is not sustained through systole.

The parasternal lift may be augmented by left atrial enlargement. The atrium is behind the right ventricle, and pushes it forward when enlarged. A rare patient with severe mitral regurgitation and left atrial enlargement may have a late-systolic parasternal lift in the absence of RV enlargement.

Emphysema changes the position of the heart in the chest. There is clockwise rotation, and the left ventricle is more posterior. The heart appears to hang vertically on the chest x-ray. The PMI that is felt in the subxyphoid region comes from the right ventricle, not the left. A forceful and sustained apex beat in this position may reflect RV hypertrophy secondary to pulmonary hypertension (*cor pulmonale*).

Heart Sounds

CHF usually has little effect on the first or second heart sounds (S_1 and S_2). With advanced heart failure and severely depressed cardiac output, the intensity of both sounds may be diminished. An especially loud S_1 may be an early finding of mitral valve stenosis, pointing to this as a cause of CHF. Similarly, an absent A_2 may indicate severe calcific aortic stenosis in an elderly patient. The rigid valve eventually stops moving, and A_2 disappears. To detect this, listen in both the pulmonic and aortic areas. P_2 is audible at the left sternal border but not to the right of the sternum. Thus, an absent S_2 at the right base indicates an immobile and probably stenotic aortic valve.

Gallops

These are low pitched sounds. The best way to hear a soft gallop is to concentrate on the segment of the cardiac cycle where it should be found. Thus, to hear an S_3, listen to the space just after S_2, ignoring all other cardiac sounds. Ask yourself, "is anything there?" If there is a soft thud, you are probably hearing the S_3. Occasionally, the gallop is something you "feel" rather than hear. If you are convinced there is no sound in that space, there is no gallop.

Both LV gallops are best heard at the apex. They are soft and may be more audible with the patient rolled to the left side. The room must be quiet. Because the sounds are low pitched, use the bell of the stethoscope, taking care not to press too firmly (which would, by tensing the underlying skin, make it work like the diaphragm). The S_3 may be localized, and you must carefully survey the apex and areas close to it. It may be hard to hear gallops in the patient with a thick chest wall. In such cases, the S_4 may be easier to hear over the sternum (bone conduction providing an aid). The timing of gallops is easier with a hand on the brachial pulse to identify systole. The S_4 is a presystolic sound and the S_3, an early diastolic ("protodiastolic") sound.

Think for a moment about the significance of gallops and the quality of the apical impulse. They are the physical findings that give you direct information about the state of the ventricle. Murmurs get a lot of attention, but they do not tell us much about the severity of disease. The gallops do just that: They tell us about ventricular size, function, and compliance.

S_3 Gallop: Big Flabby Ventricle ("Volume" Overload) The low-pitched vibration in early diastole comes from rapid ventricular filling. The mechanism is related to both high flow and the recipient ventricle being dilated and compliant. Any condition that causes ventricular dilatation and low cardiac output (with compensatory volume overload) may cause an S_3. It is the hallmark finding of cardiomyopathy. When an S_3 develops after myocardial infarction, it indicates substantial injury and worse prognosis.

S_4 Gallop: Stiff, Noncompliant Ventricle ("Pressure" Overload) This gallop at the end of diastole corresponds to elevation of the ventricular end-diastolic pressure and the A wave of the precordial impulse (Fig. 1.8). It may be called the "atrial gallop," because atrial contraction pushing the last increment of blood into a stiff ventricle generates the sound. The S_4 is absent when there is no atrial kick (e.g., atrial fibrillation, ventricular pacing, nodal or ventricular rhythms, or complete heart block). Any increase in ventricular stiffness may cause an S_4, including ventricular hypertrophy, infiltrative disease, and ischemia.

Note that I have referred to "ventricular" rather than "left ventricular" gallops. RV disease may produce gallop sounds, best heard over the left parasternal area. They may be subxyphoid in the patient with obstructive lung disease. RV gallops are augmented by inspiration (increased venous return and flow to the right ventricle). I have had little luck hearing the right-sided S_3 gallop; look for it with tricuspid regurgitation and isolated right

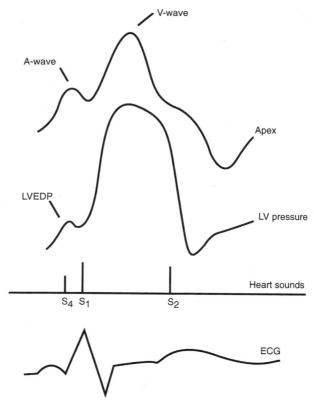

FIGURE 1.8. The contour of the apical impulse (top tracing) mirrors the LV pressure tracing. Just before ventricular systole, atrial contraction causes a small rise in LV pressure that is measured as the LV end-diastolic pressure (LVEDP). This is elevated in conditions that increase LV stiffness. It makes sense; the atrium is kicking into a ventricle that has higher pressure during diastole (it is stiff when it should be relaxed). When the apical A wave is greater than 15% of the total apical excursion, it is palpable as a shudder or glitch on the upstroke of the impulse. This is a reliable indicator of elevated LVEDP and is audible as the S_4 gallop.

heart failure. The right-sided S_4 that accompanies pulmonary hypertension is easier to hear (note the parallel with LV disease: Volume overload causes the S_3; pressure overload, the S_4).

When the heart rate is fast, it may be impossible to determine whether the gallop occurs early or late in diastole. An occasional patient with ventricular dilatation may also have increased stiffness and thus have both S_3 and S_4 gallops that are fused when heart rate is elevated. In both cases, the patient is said to have a "summation" gallop. A "gallop rhythm" refers to this combination of sounds when the rate is high (it sounds like a galloping horse).

Heart Murmurs

A loud murmur may indicate that the cause of heart failure is valvular disease (see Chapter 2). On the other hand, ventricular dilation tends to distort the orientation of the papillary muscles, and this may cause mild tricuspid or mitral regurgitation. The resulting systolic murmur is usually soft. In most cases the mildly leaking valve does not aggravate ventricular dysfunction.

Laboratory Examination

In addition to the history and physical examination, all patients suspected of having CHF should routinely have the following studies: complete blood count and urinalysis; serum chemistries, including electrolytes, renal function tests, liver function tests, albumin and thyroid function studies (especially over age 65 years or if in atrial fibrillation), chest x-ray, electrocardiogram (ECG), and echocardiogram with Doppler flow studies. These tests are used to confirm the diagnosis of CHF, to rule out specific causes of heart failure such as occult valvular disease (Table 1.5), and to exclude conditions that may aggravate CHF.

If the echocardiogram is technically inadequate (often a problem with large patients or those with emphysema), a *radionuclide angiogram (RNA)*, also called a MUGA scan, may be used to measure LVEF (Box 1.1). Red blood cells from the patient are labeled with an isotope, and the cells are reinjected. This "blood pool label" allows scanning over the heart during peak systole and peak diastole. The math is simple: If there are 100,000 counts from the left ventricle at end-diastole and 50,000 counts at peak systole, the LVEF is 50%. This test and the echocardiogram can also be used to assess LV regional wall motion. A segmental or "regional" wall motion abnormality suggests coronary artery disease and infarction, whereas global hypokinesis is more consistent with idiopathic dilated cardiomyopathy.

Coronary artery disease should be excluded, especially in younger patients with CHF and no apparent cause. The ECG usually has Q waves indicating prior infarction, but not always.

TABLE 1.5. **Studies Useful in the Initial Evaluation of Patients with Suspected Congestive Heart Failure**

Laboratory Study	Clinical Issue(s)
Complete blood count	Anemia (may aggrevate CHF; exclude high output failure)
Serum chemistry profile	Electrolyte disturbances Diabetes mellitus Renal insufficiency Hypoproteinemia
Thyroid function tests	Hyper/hypothyroidism
Urinalysis	Proteinuria (nephrotic syndrome, acute glomerulonephritis—both causes of edema)
ECG	Myocardial infarction Ventricular hypertrophy Incessant tachycardia (arrhythmia)
Chest x-ray	Confirm congestion as the cause of dyspnea (especially important when there is obstructive lung disease) Pulmonary infiltrates/fibrosis Presence of pleural effusion Cardiomegaly
Echocardiogram	Differentiate systolic vs. diastolic dysfunction Document LV dysfunction and chamber size Wall motion abnormalities (coronary artery disease as etiology) Valvular abnormalities Pericardial effusion Intracardiac masses

When the index of suspicion is low (e.g., no coronary risk factors or suggestive symptoms), a perfusion scan may be adequate (Chapter 4). When there is uncertainty or when coronary disease seems likely, go directly to coronary angiography.

Treatment

An approach to treatment of CHF caused by systolic dysfunction is outlined in Table 1.6. The nonpharmacologic measures should be adopted in every case. Most patients benefit from modest fluid restriction, drinking only when thirsty. Our heart failure clinic advises strict fluid restriction (less than 2000 mL/day) for those requiring at least 80 mg furosemide per day to control congestion or for patients with serum sodium ≤ 140 mEq/dL. We recommend continued aerobic exercise even for those with moderate to severe symptoms. Abstinence from alcohol is critical for those

TABLE 1.6. Ancillary Diagnostic Testing for CHF

Diagnostic Study/Laboratory Studies	Indication/Suspected Etiology	Comment
Serum iron/ferritin	Hemochromatosis	
ACE level	Sarcoidosis	
Toxicology screening	Heavy metal toxicity/other environmental toxin	
Blood cultures	Bacterial and fungal infectious etiologies	
Viral titers	Viral myocarditis	
Sed rate, ANA, rheumatoid factor	Collagen vascular disease	
Radionuclide ventriculography	Poor-quality echocardiogram	Useful for prognostication throughout its entire range though it loses prognostic discrimination with LVEF between 15% and 25%. Potentially inaccurate in patients with atrial fibrillation. Nonischemic cardiomyopathy may show patchy perfusion abnormalities.
Stress perfusion studies	Patients with CHF, without angina but with an intermediate risk of coronary artery disease as a possible etiology	
	Determination of myocardial viability in patients who may be candidates for revascularization	
Coronary angiography	All patients with CHF and a history consistent with angina or previous myocardial infarction (with or without recurrent angina)	
	Patients with CHF and significant risk factors for coronary artery disease	

Hemodynamic monitoring ("tailored therapy")	Patients who respond poorly to initial empiric therapy (initiation of tailored therapy) Patients being evaluated for cardiac transplantation to rule out fixed pulmonary hypertension	Tailored therapy involves optimizing filling pressures and cardiac output with a combination of intravenous inotropes and vasodilators, and then substituting oral medicines.
Endomyocardial biopsy	Recent onset of congestive heart failure with rapid clinical deterioration Past or present use of specific chemotherapy Presence of systemic disease with the possible cardiac involvement	Recent data do not support the use of steroids or other immunosuppressants in the long-term treatment of viral myocarditis. However, in a situation where patient is deteriorating rapidly, many would perform endomyocardial biopsy and treat acutely with steroids if active myocarditis is demonstrated.

with dilated cardiomyopathy, and thiamine replacement should be given to alcoholics.

ACE inhibitor therapy is indicated for CHF of all levels of severity, even for those with asymptomatic LV dysfunction (LVEF < 40%). It improves survival in patients with severe CHF and retards the progression of heart failure in patients with less severe disease (Tables 1.2 and 1.7). ACE inhibitors block the conversion of angiotensin I to angiotensin II, a potent vasoconstrictor. In addition, there is decreased aldosterone secretion and downregulation of the sympathetic nervous system. They decrease *both* afterload and preload. Note that patients with advanced aortic stenosis or LV outflow tract obstruction do not benefit from ACE inhibition; their high afterload is structural, and lowering peripheral vascular resistance will not change it.

Although most of the earlier heart failure studies were performed using enalapril or captopril, the benefits of ACE inhibition are believed to be a class effect. The dose of ACE inhibitor used in most clinical trials has been relatively high, especially compared with those used commonly in clinical practice. Typically, our heart failure clinic pushes the dose until the patient has dizziness and then backs off.

The most common adverse effect of ACE inhibitors that leads to stopping the drug is idiosyncratic cough (in as many as 10%). Rarely, it responds to cough suppressants. Angiotensin II blockers may be considered when cough prevents ACE inhibitor treatment. In addition, symptomatic orthostatic hypotension, worsening renal function, and hyperkalemia may occur with ACE inhibition. Angioedema can be mild to severe and, if encountered, requires discontinuation of ACE inhibitors with no further rechallenge. ACE inhibitors are contraindicated in pregnancy because of significant fetal and neonatal morbidity and mortality.

Hyponatremia, and Practical Tips when Starting ACE Inhibitor Therapy

It is common for patients with CHF to have depressed serum sodium. This is not the result of diuretic therapy but instead reflects elevated plasma renin activity. Those with low sodium are particularly sensitive to ACE inhibitors and may have postural hypotension when the drug is started. To avoid this, begin treatment with a lower dose than usual (e.g., captopril 6.25 mg twice a day). Remember that volume depletion increases the chance of symptomatic hypotension when starting any vasodilator. A "diuretic holiday"—holding furosemide for a couple days—before starting the ACE inhibitor may help the patient with borderline low blood pressure or when you feel that the patient is "dry." It is particularly useful when the serum sodium is below 140 mEq/dL.

Diuretics are required by most patients with CHF. Note that diuresis—a reduction in ventricular preload—does not improve ventricular function (on the contrary, it moves the patient down and to the left on the ventricular function curve; Fig. 1.4). But it is critical for the management of congestion.

Loop diuretics are used initially because of their potency. Potassium-sparing diuretics such as spironolactone (an aldosterone antagonist) are, in general, weak diuretics and do not work when given alone. Recent studies indicate a specific cardiac benefit of aldosterone inhibition (possibly with prevention of aldosterone-mediated myocardial fibrosis), and we now prescribe it routinely. In addition to its potassium-sparing effects, 50 mg spironolactone given daily has been shown to raise serum magnesium 13%.

CHF CAUSED BY DIASTOLIC DYSFUNCTION ___

Diastolic dysfunction is responsible for about one third of all CHF. Although it is possible to have diastolic failure of the right ventricle, most with diastolic dysfunction have left heart failure, and peripheral edema is unusual. By definition, patients with diastolic heart failure have normal LV systolic function. LVEF is normal or even high (the left ventricle is "hyperdynamic"). However, myocardial relaxation is impaired and/or passive stiffness is increased. Because of this increase in stiffness, the left ventricle does not fill adequately at normal pressures, so there is inadequate preload (myocardial fiber length) and low stroke volume.

Diastolic dysfunction is commonly missed as the mechanism of CHF, and we frequently see patients who are being inappropriately treated with digoxin. It is important to recognize diastolic CHF because the approach to treatment is different and the prognosis is better. The 5-year mortality for systolic heart failure is

TABLE 1.7. Drug Therapy for CHF Caused by Systolic Dysfunction

Drug Class (Preferred Agents)	Action	Comment
Diuretics	Relieve congestion, and reduce preload (and thus do not augment LV function)	Monitor serum potassium and magnesium. If the loop diuretic alone is not enough, add a thiazide (hydrochloro-thiazide is as good as metolazone). Consider spironolactone if hypokalemia is a problem. Torsemide or bumetanide may be better absorbed than furosemide when there is splanchnic congestion.
Digoxin	Increases contractility	Randomized trials showed no survival benefit, but definite symptomatic improvement and less frequent hospitalization. Use it when the patient has symptoms despite optimal ACE inhibition. Monitor levels to avoid toxicity.
ACE inhibitor	Blocks the formation of angiotensin II, a potent vasoconstrictor. Vasodilates and thus reduces afterload.	The mainstay of therapy: improves symptoms and survival and retards the progression of LV dysfunction. All drugs in this class are effective, with none shown to be superior. Most effective at high dose.
β-Adrenergic blockers (nonselective agents work best, and carvedilol is the current drug of choice)	Chronic beta stimulation increases afterload, may provoke ischemia, and may have a direct toxic effect. Beta blockade blunts this.	Carvedilol has primary vasodilating effects in addition to being a nonselective beta-blocker. Must start with a tiny dose and slowly increase it (over a few months). Temporary worsening of symptoms is common. Clinical trials showed improved survival.
Angiotensin II blockers	Action similar to ACE inhibitor, but does not cause cough.	One small study showed better survival with losartan when compared with captopril. There are fewer side effects with the A-II blockers. Large trials are pending.

Calcium channel blockers	Vasodilate and thus have the potential to reduce afterload	Studies of amlodipine showed improved symptoms, and a nonsignificant drop in mortality. Larger trials pending. We use it to control hypertension when ACE inhibitors are not enough. Consider it for CHF plus resistant angina.
Intravenous dobutamine	Increases contractility and cardiac output	Can be given at home. Intermittent therapy may be adequate (a 6-hour infusion 2–3 times each week).
Ultrafiltration	Reduces vascular volume	For use in end-stage CHF when the patient is unresponsive to diuretics—palliative care.
Anticoagulation (warfarin)	To prevent peripheral embolization	No clinical trial has supported routine anticoagulation for those in sinus rhythm with LV dysfunction. Definitely anticoagulate if there has been an embolic event, or for atrial fibrillation. Most start warfarin if the echo shows LV thrombus.
High-risk coronary revascularization	Prevention of further injury, possible restoration of hibernating myocardium	Tests of myocardial viability useful (Chapter 4).
Cardiac transplantation		5-year survival rates of 70–80% possible. Substantial morbidity with chronic immunosuppression, and donors are limited (there are organs available for 1/5 of those who would benefit).

about 50%, for diastolic CHF about 25%, and for age-matched control subjects without CHF about 5%. The mortality risk with both forms of CHF is higher with advanced age and coronary artery disease.

Any cardiac illness that provokes LVH may cause diastolic heart failure. The most common of these is hypertension, a comorbidity in about half of those with diastolic dysfunction. Others include aortic stenosis and hypertrophic cardiomyopathy. Myocardial ischemia also causes diastolic dysfunction, because myocardial relaxation is an energy-requiring process. An occasional patient presents with exertional dyspnea as a manifestation of ischemia. Transient diastolic dysfunction may be the mechanism of this "anginal equivalent"; there is pulmonary congestion but no pain. In others with chronic diastolic dysfunction, transient ischemia may aggravate symptoms.

Diastolic heart failure is a condition of advanced age. Old people get stiff hearts as well as stiff joints. It is more common in women as well. In one study, diastolic failure accounted for 10% of all cases of CHF at age 60 years but for 50% at age 80 years. In nursing homes, where the ratio of women to men is 7:1, more than half of those with CHF have diastolic failure.

Pathophysiology

Ventricular filling between heartbeats determines preload, so *diastolic* dysfunction is about *preload*. Students are often confused by "preload," because we describe it using two different measurements. In reality, preload is the length of the muscle fiber just before contraction, or in the case of the intact heart, the volume of the left ventricle at the end of diastole. But it is hard to measure LV volume and impossible to monitor it continuously. For this reason, you never see end-diastolic volume on the abscissa of the LV function (Starling) curve (Fig. 1.1). Instead, we substitute the more easily monitored end-diastolic pressure. That works most of the time, because diastolic pressure and volume are proportional (Fig. 1.2).

The problem is that a fall in LV compliance (diastolic dysfunction) changes the pressure–volume relation. Higher pressure is needed to generate a given LV volume (Fig. 1.2). This, in turn, changes the LV function curve. In such cases, the ventricle must operate with a much higher than normal diastolic pressure to maintain stroke volume and cardiac output. Recall that during diastole the mitral valve is open, so the left ventricle is in contact with the left atrium and pulmonary capillary bed. Thus, the high diastolic pressure is transmitted to the lungs, and congestion results. (The system generates high diastolic pressures via the neurohormonal and renal responses to low cardiac output, which lead to volume expansion—the same response to inadequate renal perfusion that occurs with systolic dysfunction.)

The contribution of atrial contraction to stroke volume is critical when there is diastolic dysfunction. Contraction of the atria at the end of diastole provides the last increment of ventricular filling, increasing preload and thus stroke volume (Fig. 1.3). When atrial contraction is lost (with atrial fibrillation or ventricular pacing), preload falls and with it, stroke volume. The simple and interesting experiment that defined the contribution of the atrial kick to cardiac output is illustrated in Figure 1.3. A person with normal diastolic function may have a 10% drop in cardiac output when atrial contraction is bypassed with ventricular pacing. But another with diastolic dysfunction may have cardiac output fall 25% or more with loss of the atrial kick. Atrial contraction contributes to preload, and patients with diastolic dysfunction are said to be "preload dependent."

Consider these two clinical examples of diastolic dysfunction. 1) A patient with aortic stenosis and LVH may have a big drop in blood pressure with development of atrial fibrillation. If hypotension is severe and the patient appears to be in shock, the atrial fibrillation is a medical emergency and requires immediate dc cardioversion. 2) Another patient with diastolic heart failure has a cardiac catheterization. The contrast agent functions as an osmotic diuretic, and severe hypotension may develop in the hours after catheterization with volume depletion. In such cases we pay especially careful attention to hydration for 12 hours after the procedure.

History and Physical Examination

Diastolic heart failure may be mild, with effort intolerance or dyspnea with exertion the only symptoms. Occasionally, diastolic dysfunction is diagnosed from the echocardiogram in asymptomatic patients with hypertension.

At the other end of the spectrum is the syndrome called "flash pulmonary edema," or pulmonary edema of abrupt onset. This may occur in a person with no prior history of CHF or heart disease and without gradually increasing exertional dyspnea or orthopnea before. It illustrates an important clinical feature of diastolic CHF, the narrow window between volume overload (congestion) and depletion (hypotension). Even a small increase in volume, perhaps due to increased salt intake, may precipitate pulmonary congestion. By that same token, flash pulmonary edema usually responds to modest diuresis using lower doses of furosemide than are needed with systolic CHF.

Features of the history that point to diastolic dysfunction as the cause of CHF include advanced age, hypertension, and female gender. Both the history and physical examination should screen for other conditions that may cause LVH such as aortic stenosis or hypertrophic subaortic stenosis. Look carefully for any evidence of coronary artery disease. Myocardial relaxation is an active energy-requiring process, and ischemia has an immediate negative effect.

Most patients with diastolic CHF have just pulmonary congestion; right heart failure is unusual. Thus, jugular venous distension and peripheral edema are not usually present. The physical findings of left heart congestion are typical.

The cardiac examination may allow you to differentiate diastolic from systolic failure at the bedside. With diastolic CHF the heart is usually small, so the PMI is in the mid-clavicular line. It is not diffuse and sustained. If there is LVH it may be forceful. There is no S_3 gallop. Instead, increased LV diastolic stiffness causes an S_4 gallop, the result of the atrium forcing blood into the stiff ventricle at the end of diastole.

An even neater physical finding is a palpable S_4, the *apical A wave* (Fig. 1.8). To detect the A wave, have the patient roll to the left and carefully feel the apical impulse. Normally the upstroke of the PMI is smooth. The A wave is felt as a glitch or shudder in the upstroke. Practice feeling for it in those with hypertension and LVH; it is not that subtle a finding. Describing an apical A wave is a sophisticated physical diagnosis maneuver (and very cool). More importantly, it is the most specific physical finding for increased LV stiffness, and its presence reliably indicates elevated LV diastolic pressure. Remember that the A wave and S_4

gallop disappear with atrial fibrillation and the loss of atrial contraction (medical residents *always* ask students if they hear the S_4 in patients with atrial fibrillation—do not be fooled).

Laboratory Examination

There are just two things needed to make the diagnosis of diastolic failure. The first is to establish the diagnosis of CHF. A chest x-ray showing congestion that subsequently responds to diuresis is adequate evidence.

The second step is documentation of LVEF. If the LVEF is above 40%, then it is diastolic heart failure. That is the criterion used in most studies of diastolic dysfunction; in practice, most patients have normal or even hyperdynamic LV contraction, and the ventricle is small.

Supporting evidence includes LVH on the ECG or echocardiogram. Remember that only 50% of those with increased LV thickness on the echo meet ECG criteria for LVH. Diastolic dysfunction is about abnormal LV filling, and the echo-Doppler study allows assessment of flow across the mitral valve during diastole (Fig. 1.9). Normally, flow into the ventricle is highest in early diastole, but with increased LV stiffness the velocity of flow after atrial contraction—the A wave—increases.

The echocardiogram may not be technically adequate to assess LV size and function (in a setting of obesity or emphysema). The other noninvasive tool for measuring LVEF is RNA. Using the "first-pass" technique, the RNA can also provide information about LV filling. In the absence of CHF, echo-Doppler findings of abnormal diastolic filling identify preclinical diastolic dysfunction, strong evidence for treatment aimed at regression of LVH.

It is important to exclude ischemic heart disease, especially for a younger patient. In addition to controlling symptoms caused by transient ischemia in an already stiff ventricle, you want to intervene before the patient has a myocardial infarction. Combined systolic and diastolic dysfunction—often the case with ischemic cardiomyopathy—is the worst of all possible worlds. In the absence of anginal symptoms and risk factors, a screening perfusion study may be adequate. If the symptoms are suggestive, consider cardiac catheterization. This is also useful when there is uncertainty about the diagnosis (is CHF causing the patient's symptoms?). A normal LV end-diastolic pressure at

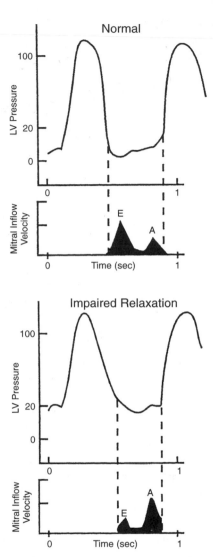

FIGURE 1.9. The effect of impaired LV relaxation on LV pressure (measured at cardiac catheterization) and flow across the mitral valve (measured from the echo-Doppler study). Normally, maximal flow into the ventricle occurs in early diastole, the E wave. With impaired relaxation in early diastole, atrial contraction produces a higher flow velocity, and the A wave is larger than the V wave. Note that with the stiffer ventricle the LV diastolic pressure is higher.

rest and with arm exercise in the catheterization lab is proof of normal diastolic function.

Treatment

Unlike systolic heart failure, there have been no large clinical trials of therapy for diastolic failure. The strategy outlined in Table 1.8 is a reasonable approach based on experience and the pathophysiology of the illness and should be considered in all patients.

Congestion is relieved by lowering preload. Small doses of furosemide are usually sufficient, because the pressure volume curve is steep, and there is a narrow difference between congestion and volume depletion. It is common to overshoot with diuretics. We usually begin with 20 mg furosemide daily and carefully titrate the dose. Stable patients may be controlled with 12.5 to 25 mg hydrochlorothiazide per day. Nitrates may also be used to reduce preload, especially when there is ischemia. Again, start with a low dose, 5 to 10 mg isosorbide dinitrate three times a day.

Reducing blood pressure has an immediate benefit, because the excessive afterload of hypertension slows relaxation. Over the long run, control of blood pressure leads to regression of LVH and improved diastolic function. ACE inhibitors appear to be the most effective for regression of hypertrophy, and they may have a direct myocardial effect. Calcium channel blockers, beta-blockers, and centrally acting sympatholytic agents also work. Early data suggest a role for aldosterone antagonists (spironolactone).

Tachycardia is a major problem when there is diastolic disease. The duration of systole is constant at all heart rates. At rapid rates, the total duration of diastole thus declines, and there is less time for ventricular filling. Drugs that lower the sinus rate (beta-blockers, verapamil, or diltiazem) or control the rate with atrial fibrillation (the one use for digoxin in diastolic failure) will improve exercise tolerance. Pure arterial dilators used in the absence of hypertension do lower afterload, but they also cause reflex tachycardia; the net effect may be worsening diastolic function.

I have emphasized the importance of atrial contraction in the patient with a stiff left ventricle. Unfortunately, atrial fibrillation is a common complication of diastolic failure, because there is elevation of the left atrial pressure (often called "left atrial hypertension"). Every effort should be made to restore sinus rhythm.

TABLE 1.8. The Treatment Strategy for Diastolic CHF

Goal of Treatment	Intervention/Drug	Comment
Reduce preload and congestion	Diuretics, occasionally nitrates	The LV pressure volume curve is steep with diastolic failure; small changes in volume lead to big changes in pressure. Thus, *low-dose* diuresis usually works
Treat hypertension and reduce LVH	First choice: ACE inhibitors. Calcium blockers, beta-blockers, and central alpha-blockers also work.	Short-term benefit: lower afterload favorably affects LV relaxation. Long-term benefit: regression of LVH.
Treat ischemia	Revascularization when possible. Beta blockade and calcium blockade.	Ischemia directly impairs LV relaxation. Consider an "anginal equivalent" for the patient with new onset, exertional dyspnea with an anginal pattern.
Lower heart rate to 60–70 beats/min	Beta-blockers, verapamil and diltiazem	At higher heart rates, the total diastolic time is reduced, so there is less time for LV filling. These drugs may be used even when blood pressure is normal to blunt exercise-induced tachycardia.
Maintain atrial booster function	Correct atrial fibrillation.	The stiff LV is especially dependent on atrial contraction for adequate filling.
Avoid inotropes and pure arterial dilators	Avoid digoxin, hydralazine, and calcium blockers that are pure vasodilators (nifedipine).	Drugs that increase contractility also impair myocardial relaxation. Vasodilation may provoke reflex tachycardia.

SUGGESTED READINGS

ACC/AHA Task Force Report. Guidelines for the evaluation and management of heart failure. JACC 1995;26:1376–1404.

Australia-New Zealand Heart Research Collaborative Group. Effects of carvedilol, a vasodilator-beta-blocker, in patients with congestive heart failure due to ischemic heart disease. Circulation 1995;92:212–219. (This and other studies of beta blockade cited below showed improved survival.)

Blake P, Paganini EP. Refractory congestive heart failure: overview and application of extracorporeal ultrafiltration. Adv Renal Replace Ther 1996;3:166–171.

Brown NJ, Vaughan DE. Angiotensin converting enzyme inhibitors. Circulation 1998;97:1411–1420. (Good review of clinical trials, a number of them cited below.)

CIBIS Investigators and Committees. A randomized trial of beta blockade and heart failure: the cardiac insufficiency bisoprolol study (CIBIS). Circulation 1994;90:1765–1772.

Cohn JN, Archibald DG, Ziesche S, et al. Effect of vasodilator therapy on mortality in chronic congestive heart failure. N Engl J Med 1986;314:1547–1556.

Cohn JN, Johnson G, Ziesche S, et al. A comparison of enalapril with hydralazine-isosorbide dinitrate in the treatment of chronic congestive heart failure. N Engl J Med 1991;325:303–310.

Cohn JN, Ziesche S, Smith R, et al. The effect of the calcium antagonist felodipine as supplementary vasodilator therapy in patients with chronic heart failure treated with enalapril V-HeFT III. Circulation 1997;96:856–862.

CONSENSUS Trial Study Group. Effects of enalapril on mortality in severe congestive heart failure: results of the Cooperative North Scandinavian Enalapril Survival Study (CONSENSUS). N Engl J Med 1987;216:1409–1419.

Conti CR. Assessing ventricular function. Clin Cardiol 2000; 23:557–558. (Compares imaging techniques, and concludes that "the best buys for the money are the combination of physical examination, chest x-ray, electrocardiogram and cardiac ultrasound.")

Costanzo MR. Current status of heart transplantation. Curr Opin Cardiol 1996;11:161–172.

DeMaria AN, Blanchard D. The hemodynamic basis of diastology. J Am Coll Cardiol 1999;34:1659–1662. (A good review of echo-Doppler techniques for evaluating LV diastolic function.)

Digitalis Investigators Group. The effect of digoxin on mortality and morbidity in patients with heart failure. N Engl J Med 1997;336:525–531. (The key is that digoxin did not increase mortality, as have other inotropic agents. There was improvement in symptoms and reduced hospitalization.)

Eichhorn EJ, Bristow MR. Medical therapy can improve the biological properties of the chronically failing heart: a new era in the treatment of heart failure. Circulation 1996;94:2285–2287.

Ho KKL, Anderson KM, Kannel WB, et al. Survival after the onset of congestive heart failure in Framingham Heart Study subjects. Circulation 1993;88:107–152.

Ho KKL, Pinsky JL, Kannel WB, Levy D. The epidemiology of heart failure: the Framingham Study. JACC 1993;22:6A–20A.

Hunter JJ, Chien KR. Signaling pathways for cardiac hypertorphy and failure. N Engl J Med 1999;341:1276–1284. (The molecular biology for cardiac dilation and hypertrophy.)

Krum H. New and emerging pharmacologic strategies in the management of chronic heart failure. Clin Cardiol 2000;23:724–730.

(Review of ongoing clinical trials of endothelin inhibition, cytokine antagonists, and natriuretic peptide augmentation.)

Mason JW, O'Connell JB, Herskowitz A, et al. A clinical trial of immunosuppressive therapy for myocarditis. N Engl J Med 1995;333:269–276.

Packer M, et al. for the ATLAS Study Group. Comparative effects of low and high doses of lisinopril on morbidity and mortality in chronic heart failure. Circulation 1999;100:2312–2318. (Patients randomized to a higher dose group [average above 30 mg/day] did better than others on 5 mg/day.)

Packer M, O'Connor CM, Ghali JK, et al. Effect amlodipine on morbidity and mortality in severe chronic heart failure. N Engl J Med 1996;335:1107. (The pure vasodilator and calcium blocker is an effective afterload reducer, but it's clinical effects do not match ACE inhibition.)

Pitt B, Zannad F, Remme WJ. The effect of spironolactone on morbidity and mortality in patients with severe heart failure. N Engl J Med 1999;341:709–717. (There was a 30% reduction in death during 24 months' follow-up with spironolactone 25 mg/day.)

Segal B, Martinez R, Meures FA, et al. Randomized trial of losartan vs captopril in patients over 65 with heart failure (Evaluation of Losartan in the Elderly Study, ELITE). Lancet 1997;349:747–753. (The angiotensin-II blockers are as effective as ACE inhibitors.)

Singh SN, Fletcher RD, Fisher SH, et al. Amiodarone in patients with congestive heart failure and asymptomatic ventricular arrhythmia. N Engl J Med 1995;333:77–85. (Amiodarone is the only antiarrhythmic agent that does not increase the risk of sudden death in patients with severe LV dysfunction.)

SOLVED Investigators. Effect of enalapril on mortality and the development of heart failure in asymptomatic patients with reduced left ventricular ejection fractions. N Engl J Med 1992; 307:685–692. (Based on this study, do not wait for symptoms to develop, but treat all with LV dysfunction.)

SOLVED Investigators. Effect of enalapril on survival in patients with reduced left ventricular ejection fraction and congestive heart failure. N Engl J Med 1991;325:293–300.

Starling RC. Radical alternatives to transplantation. Curr Opin Cardiol 1997;12:166–178.

Stevenson WG, Stevenson LW, Middlekouff HR, et al. Improving survival for patients with advanced heart failure: a study of 737 consecutive patients. JACC 1995;26:1417–1425.

Sugrue DD, Rodeheffer RJ, Codd MD, et al. The clinical course of idiopathic dilated cardiomyopathy: a population-based study. Ann Intern Med 1992;117:117–127.

Waagstein F, Bristow MR, Swedberg K, et al. Beneficial effects of metoprolol in idiopathic dilated cardiomyopathy. Lancet 1993; 342:141–148.

Wiese J. The abdominojugular reflux sign. Am J Med 2000;109:59–61. (The sign is not specific to any one disorder and is a reflection of a right ventricle that cannot accommodate venous return. RV infarction and constrictive pericarditis are possible causes, and left heart failure may cause it when the pulmonary wedge pressure is above 15. Cardiac tamponade does not cause it.)

Williams RS. Apoptosis and heart failure. N Engl J Med 1999;341:759–760.

CHAPTER 2

Valvular Heart Disease

Valvular heart disease is, in a sense, the applied cardiac physiology laboratory. To understand it, you must develop a feel for cardiac loading (preload and afterload). When you approach the patient with a murmur, ask yourself the following questions. They may seem simplistic—and are simple—but if you focus on them while studying valvular disease, you will memorize less and understand more:

1. What chamber is most affected by the valve lesion (Table 2.1)?
2. What is the effect on the chamber? Does the lesion change preload, afterload, or contractility, and is there hypertrophy or dilatation?
3. What physical findings might be expected with these changes in chamber size and function? In particular, what happens to the apical impulse, and which gallop should you hear?
4. What diagnostic study will identify altered chamber size and function and thus define the "hemodynamic significance" of the lesion?
5. What changes in left ventricle size and function necessitate valve surgery, and how will surgery affect function?

MITRAL STENOSIS

For practical purposes, mitral stenosis (MS) may be equated with rheumatic heart disease (RHD). All patients with RHD have scarring of the mitral valve. This has a typical appearance on the echocardiogram, and you may therefore use the echo to diagnose or exclude RHD.

Mitral stenosis has become an unusual illness in the West because of aggressive treatment of streptococcal infection. It is common in less-developed countries. In rural Latin America or

India, RHD has a more aggressive course, with symptomatic MS and other valvular disease developing at a younger age. In the United States, young people seldom have hemodynamically significant MS. The usual history is rheumatic fever in the early teens and then onset of symptoms or atrial fibrillation when the patient is 40 to 60 years old.

I have seen a number of patients older than 70 years, usually women, with refractory congestive heart failure who had MS as an unexpected finding on the echocardiogram. The murmur may be soft or absent because of depressed cardiac output and reduced flow across the stenosed valve. And a heavily calcified, immobile valve may not generate an opening snap. In elderly patients, pulmonary congestion may not be a prominent feature of the illness; the chief complaint may be fatigue or weight loss. This is one reason an echocardiogram is justified in older patients with vague nonspecific symptoms (a screen for occult valvular or myocardial disease).

Pathophysiology, History, and Physical Examination

One of my teachers told us that "mitral stenosis is a disease of the lungs." The blocked valve causes pressure overload of the left atrium (LA), and LA dilatation (Table 2.1). The increased pressure in the LA is transmitted to the pulmonary capillary bed. Dyspnea on exertion, fatigue (due to limited cardiac output), and winter bronchitis are the usual symptoms, and they may be insidious in onset. A middle-aged nurse with known MS for years called this winter to get an antibiotic for a "chest cold she couldn't shake." She and her family doctor were concerned she might be developing asthma. But with questioning she admitted that her exercise tolerance had gradually worsened over the previous 4 to 6 months. This is the typical, slowly evolving story. Patients are often unaware just how bad they feel until symptoms are relieved by valve surgery.

With time, most patients with LA enlargement caused by mitral valve disease develop atrial fibrillation.

The left ventricle is not overloaded with MS. The stenosed valve "protects" the left ventricle, which is small and contracts normally (unless there is associated cardiomyopathy, which may complicate rheumatic fever). Dyspnea is the result of left ventric-

TABLE 2.1. Overview of Valvular Heart Disease

Lesion	Chamber/Effect	Indications for Surgery
Mitral stenosis (MS)	Left atrial pressure overload, LA dilatation. LV preload is low (MS impedes LV filling), even though vascular volume is high. There is pulmonary congestion, but with sparing of the LV there is no gallop.	There is no risk of LV injury, so surgery may be based on symptoms (pulmonary congestion, fatigue).
Acute mitral regurgitation (MR)	LA and LV volume overload (LV preload is high). Ventricular pressure is transmitted to the lungs, and there is a V wave on the wedge pressure tracing. With acute onset there is no time for either LA or LV dilatation.	Severe congestion necessitates urgent surgery in most cases.
Chronic MR	LA and LV volume overload and dilatation; LV preload is high. The LA "gives," absorbing the LV pressure wave, so there is no V wave on the wedge tracing. Eventually there is LV contractile dysfunction. S_3 gallop reflects LV volume overload, dilatation, and dysfunction.	Net LV afterload is low (see text), falsely elevating LVEF. The LV is not as good as it seems and may worsen after surgery (which raises afterload). Surgery is needed with depression of LVEF or a rise in LV end-systolic dimension above 4.5 cm, even in the absence of symptoms.
Aortic stenosis (AS)	LV pressure overload (a pure afterload condition). S_4 gallop and apical A wave with LVH. Possible loss of A_2 with a heavily calcified valve.	Valve replacement reduces afterload, so LV function improves after surgery. The usual indication for surgery is symptoms (which may be subtle, see text).
Aortic regurgitation (AR)	LV volume overload. Afterload is increased as well, so there is both dilatation and hypertrophy (see text). Wide pulse pressure is due to peripheral vasodilatation.	As with MR, do not delay repair until CHF develops. A fall in LVEF or rise in end-systolic dimension above 4.5 cm are indications for surgery.
Tricuspid regurgitation (TR)	RV and RA volume overload. The RV pressure wave is transmitted to the jugular veins (V wave) and the liver (which is pulsatile). Think of TR when there is right-sided congestion (edema).	TR usually complicates left heart failure or mitral valve disease. The tricuspid valve may be repaired if TR remains severe after mitral valve repair.

LA, left atrium; LV, left ventricle; RA, right atrial.

ular (LV) inflow obstruction; LV preload is low. On the other hand, high left atrial pressure and low cardiac output mimic congestive heart failure caused by LV dysfunction. The neurohumoral response to low cardiac output is the same (see Chapter 1).

Now we have the information needed to understand the cardiac examination. The position and quality of the apical impulse are normal, and there is no gallop (reflecting a normal left ventricle). There is a diastolic murmur across the stenosed valve, and it is low pitched. It is best heard at the apex, because the stenotic jet is "aimed" at the apex of the left ventricle.

The Opening Snap

This interesting physical finding is generated by movement of the rigid calcified valve. It is a high-pitched sound that is easy to hear at the apex, just after S_2. With more severe stenosis the opening snap occurs earlier, and an S_2–opening snap interval less than 0.11 seconds indicates severe stenosis. Measuring this interval using the phonocardiogram was the best noninvasive test for severity of MS in the days before echocardiography. That test is no longer used, but you can estimate the S_2–opening snap interval at the bedside using an old-fashioned diagnostic trick to estimate this brief time interval. When you say the words, the interval between the letters b and l in "blah" is 0.10 seconds and between the b and t in "butter" is 0.14 seconds. Admittedly low-tech, but it works, and making an accurate guess about the severity of a valvular lesion is still great sport for clinicians.

Diagnostic Tests

The electrocardiogram (ECG) shows left atrial enlargement, usually with the "P mitrale" pattern (Fig. 2.1). Notching of the P waves in leads II, III, and aVF appears more common with pressure overload of the LA rather than biphasic P's in V_1. Another common ECG pattern is atrial fibrillation.

Left atrial enlargement causes straightening of the left heart border on the chest x-ray and a double density at the right heart border where the left atrial shadow is just inside the right atrial shadow. There may be Kerley B lines with pulmonary congestion (thickened pulmonary lymphatics and septae).

The echocardiogram demonstrates rheumatic deformity of the valve, reduced valve mobility and, with long-standing disease, calcification of the leaflets. All patients have left atrial enlargement. There are three methods for measuring the severity of MS using the echo-Doppler study. The first is visualization of the valve in cross-section and measuring the size of the opening.

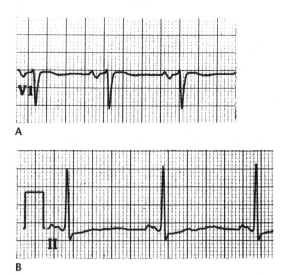

FIGURE 2.1. Left atrial abnormality. Two ECG findings may be used to make the diagnosis. (A) Biphasic P wave in lead V_1; the negative deflection should be 1 mm deep and wide. (B) Broad notched P wave in one of the limb leads, most commonly II, III, or aVF (as the P wave vector is aimed inferiorly).

Two Doppler measures of severity come from flow velocity across the mitral valve. Flow velocity, in meters per second, is proportional to stenosis (this is analogous to increased flow at the end of a garden hose when the nozzle is tightened). In addition, flow velocity remains high for a longer time with stenosis, decaying at the very end of diastole. The "pressure half-time" is a measure of the time to decay of the flow velocity curve and is proportional to severity of stenosis.

Cardiac catheterization is seldom needed for evaluation of the valve but is usually recommended to exclude coronary artery disease in older patients. The valve gradient is measured using catheters in the pulmonary artery and left ventricle (Fig. 2.2).

Treatment

Asymptomatic patients in sinus rhythm require only antibiotic prophylaxis for infective endocarditis. For mild symptoms, diuretics lower left atrial pressure and relieve congestion. Because LV function is normal, there is no role for measures to lower afterload or increase contractility.

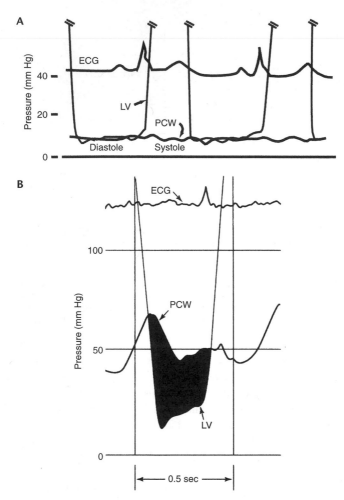

FIGURE 2.2. Pressure tracings from the cardiac catheterization laboratory. (A) Normal. The pulmonary capillary wedge (PCW) pressure is identical to left atrial pressure during diastole (there is no valve separating the pulmonary artery from the left atrium). There is no difference, or "gradient," between left atrial and LV diastolic pressure when the normal mitral valve is open. (B) Mitral stenosis. Even when the mitral valve is open during diastole, there is a pressure gradient caused by stenosis (shaded area). (Reproduced by permission from Carabello BA, Grossman W, eds. Cardiac catheterization and angiography, 3rd ed. Philadelphia: Lea & Febiger, 1986.)

Atrial fibrillation is common. Reduced flow across the mitral valve plus the enlarged LA make the risk of peripheral embolization and stroke much higher than it is with other causes of atrial fibrillation. Warfarin therapy is needed (see Chapter 6). Rate control with digoxin, beta-blockers, or calcium blockers is especially important for control of symptoms. Tachycardia reduces total diastolic time, a big problem for the patient with LV inflow obstruction who needs extra time for LV filling.

MS is a mechanical problem and eventually requires a mechanical (surgical) solution. The prognosis worsens when more than mild symptoms develop or there is pulmonary hypertension (which can be diagnosed with the echo-Doppler study). Those are the usual indications for surgery.

Recall that the left ventricle is protected. Surgery is not required prophylactically to save the left ventricle. Some authorities recommend surgery when atrial fibrillation develops and cannot be converted and maintained. In this case, correction of MS may allow the LA to shrink, restoring sinus rhythm.

When the valve is mobile and there is little calcification—often the case with younger patients—repair is possible. Closed balloon valvulotomy works well, with an average doubling of valve area that is maintained long term. Associated mitral regurgitation (MR), thrombus in the LA, and valve calcification are contraindications to balloon repair and indicate a need for surgery.

MITRAL REGURGITATION (MR) _____

Acute Mitral Regurgitation

MR after acute myocardial infarction is caused by injury of a papillary muscle, a complication reviewed in Chapter 5. Spontaneous or traumatic rupture of chordae may occur in the absence of coronary artery disease, most commonly in middle-aged men with mitral valve prolapse (MVP). The history may include a single brief episode of chest pain at the time of rupture. Over the next few days there is progressive dyspnea, and severe pulmonary congestion is apparent at the time of initial evaluation.

TABLE 2.2. Acute vs. Chronic MR

	Acute MR	Chronic MR
Etiology	Papillary muscle rupture during acute myocardial infarction or rupture of a cord in the absence of CAD (usually middle-aged men).	MVP is the most common cause (middle-aged men at highest risk). Rheumatic heart disease a rare cause in the U.S.
Chamber size (echo findings)— gallop	No time for LA or LV dilatation. Possibly an S_4 (large volume to a small noncompliant LV). Normal heart size on chest x-ray.	Marked LA and LV dilatation. S_3 (rapid filling of a large flabby LV). Big heart on chest x-ray.
Hemo-dynamics	High pulmonary wedge pressure with a prominent V wave (the small and stiff LA transmits the regurgitant wave directly to the lungs).	Wedge pressure may be normal in the absence of pulmonary congestion (the patient is still "compensated"). Small V wave as the dilated LA absorbs the regurgitant pressure wave.
Clinical history	Abrupt onset of pulmonary congestion, often new pulmonary edema	Congestion may appear late in the clinical course, and symptoms of CHF develop more slowly.
Timing of surgery	Pulmonary edema necessi-tates urgent surgery.	Any fall in LVEF or a rise in LV end-systolic size are indications for surgery, even in the absence of symptoms (see text).
Prognosis	Good after surgical repair, because dramatic symptoms usually force intervention before there is permanent LV damage.	Poor if surgery is delayed. By the time the patient is severely symptomatic, it may be too late to save the LV (see text). The patient winds up with a new valve but has dilated cardio-myopathy.

LA, left atrium; LV, left ventricle; CHF, congestive heart failure; MVP, mitral valve prolapse.

Pathophysiology, Physical Examination, and Laboratory Evaluation

Because of the rapid onset of symptoms, there is insufficient time for the LA and LV to dilate (Table 2.2). Therefore, the apical impulse is not displaced. There is no S_3 gallop, despite severe heart failure (recall that the S_3 gallop is caused by rapid filling of a big flabby left ventricle). In fact, the large volume of blood hitting the relatively small left ventricle at end-diastole may cause an S_4 gallop. A small and stiff LA is unable to "accommodate" the regurgitant wave. The marked rise in LA pressure that follows LV contraction is called the V wave (Fig. 2.3). This V wave is transmitted directly to the pulmonary capillary bed, aggravating congestive symptoms.

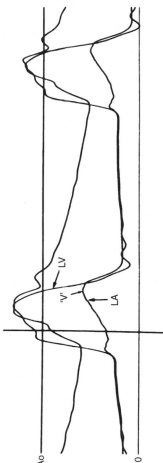

FIGURE 2.3. Simultaneous left atrial (LA), LV, and aortic (Ao) pressure tracings from a patient with *acute* MR. During LV systole, the LV pressure wave is transmitted back to the LA through the defective mitral valve and is measured as a "V" wave. In the absence of MR there is a tiny V wave caused by the slight posterior bowing of the mitral valve. With *chronic* MR the large flaccid left atrium absorbs the pressure wave and the V wave is not as prominent. (Reproduced by permission from Taylor GJ. Primary care cardiology. Boston: Blackwell Science, 1995.)

LV stroke volume and ejection fraction (EF) are high, but this is misleading because much of the ejected volume is "wasted," going to the LA rather than the aorta.

When MR is severe and symptomatic, the murmur tends to be loud, holosystolic, and harsh. I was taught that the MR murmur radiates to the axilla, but that may not be the case with acute MR. Dysfunction of the support structures for the *lateral* leaflet causes it to prolapse; this creates a "baffle" effect, aiming the regurgitant jet medially. The murmur is then heard along the left sternal border and at the base of the heart, mimicking aortic stenosis (though it does not radiate to the neck). If papillary muscle dysfunction is the etiology, the murmur may even be diamond shaped, because peak dysfunction and leak occur at peak LV pressure in mid-systole.

The echo-Doppler study documents the regurgitant jet. LA and LV size are normal. A regional wall motion abnormality suggests ischemic papillary muscle injury as the cause of MR. A "flail" mitral leaflet often is visible. Cardiac catheterization is usually performed to define coronary artery anatomy.

Treatment

Acute MR with severe pulmonary congestion is a surgical emergency. Most of these patients have damage to valve support structures, and the valve leaflets may be normal. Valve repair rather than replacement is a possibility. This has definite advantages over valve replacement. Chronic anticoagulation is unnecessary and LV function is better preserved, possibly because the papillary muscles are saved. It seems that papillary muscles contribute to overall LV performance, by tethering the LV on its long axis. With their loss there is increased ventricular volume and reduced LVEF. Even with valve replacement, current technique calls for saving the chordae rather than transecting them.

Chronic Mitral Regurgitation

RHD does not cause isolated MR. There is always MS as well, and this is evident on the echocardiogram. Isolated MR is caused by the MVP syndrome, ischemic injury of papillary muscles, LV dilatation (which changes the orientation of the papillary muscles and dilates the valve ring), or infective endocarditis.

Pathophysiology and Physical Examination

The mitral valve leak is not as severe as it is with acute MR (allowing the condition to be chronic). There is volume overload of the LA and left ventricle, and dilatation of these chambers develops slowly (Table 2.2).

The dilated LA "gives," absorbing the shock of the regurgitant jet. Thus, there is not a prominent V wave on the pulmonary wedge tracing (Fig. 2.3). The apical impulse is displaced and has a volume overload quality; it is "rocking" and occupies more than one rib interspace. There may be an S_3 gallop caused by the rapid filling wave in early diastole.

The murmur is holosystolic, extending to S_2, and audible at the apex and axilla. As with acute MR, a dysfunctional lateral leaflet may prolapse and serve as a baffle, directing the jet—and murmur—toward the base of the heart rather than the axilla. (Prolapse of the medial leaflet would baffle the jet toward the axilla.)

It is important to understand LV afterload in the setting of MR (Fig. 2.4). It is low, right? Normally, systemic arterial resistance constitutes the impedance to LV ejection. With MR the ventricle is able to unload into both the low-pressure LA and the higher-pressure aorta (Fig. 2.4). Net impedance to ejection, or afterload, is low. Low afterload makes it easy for the LV muscle to shorten, so LVEF is artificially high. When the mitral valve is repaired and the left ventricle can no longer dump its load into the low-pressure LA, there is a net increase in afterload. Thus, LVEF may decline after correction of MR. As noted, another reason for deterioration of LV function with valve replacement is loss of the papillary muscles.

For these reasons surgery for chronic MR is high risk. The quality of LV function preoperatively is overestimated, and function often declines after surgery. Unlike MS, symptoms may be an unreliable guide to therapy. By the time a patient with MR is symptomatic, irreversible LV injury may have occurred.

Timing of Surgery and Laboratory Evaluation

The best predictors of outcome are LVEF and end-systolic volume. Because LVEF is expected to decline with surgery, a preoperative LVEF < 50% is a terrible prognostic sign. Dilatation of the left ventricle during diastole is not a problem if the ventricle contracts down to a normal volume at end-systole (this, of course,

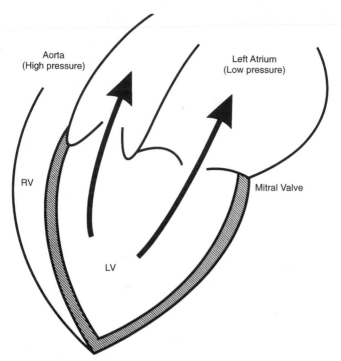

FIGURE 2.4. MR and left ventricular afterload. In the absence of MR, the ventricle empties into the aorta, a high-pressure system. But with MR the left ventricle (LV) can also empty into the low-pressure left atrium. The net afterload, or impedance to ejection, is therefore low. Repairing the valve may be expected to increase net afterload, and left ventricular function suffers. RV, right ventricle.

also indicates normal LVEF). With volume overload disease, both MR and aortic regurgitation (AR), an elevated preoperative end-systolic volume predicts higher operative mortality, more postoperative heart failure, and persistent LV enlargement after surgery.

The end-systolic transverse dimension can be substituted for LV volume. This measurement is easily and accurately obtained from the echocardiogram. When the end-systolic dimension exceeds 5 cm, there is increased risk of surgery.

Surgery is usually recommended when the end-systolic dimension reaches 4.5 cm or the LVEF falls below 55% to 60%, even when the patient has no symptoms. Asymptomatic patients have serial echocardiograms to follow these LV measurements. Follow-up Doppler studies are unnecessary, because you already know there is MR. Order the cheaper "echo without Doppler."

Choice of Valve Prosthesis

None of them is perfect. If we had a perfect valve and a risk-free operation, the timing of surgery would be easier. The choice of valves comes down to durability versus thromboembolic potential.

Tissue valves (the porcine bioprosthesis) have low thromboembolic potential, and aspirin therapy is adequate. They begin to wear out in 10 to 12 years (much earlier in growing children with more active calcium metabolism).

The more durable mechanical valves have a thromboembolic rate of three to eight events per 100 valve-years, which is substantially reduced by warfarin therapy. Warfarin carries a risk of two hemorrhagic events per 100 patient years, usually nonfatal gastrointestinal bleed. Most thromboembolic events are strokes. Thus, the evidence weighs in favor of warfarin for all with a mechanical valve. This is more important for valves in the mitral position, with a higher stroke rate than aortic valve prostheses.

Tissue valves are currently used when there is a contraindication to warfarin therapy or for the elderly where 10-year valve longevity is adequate (and anticoagulation is riskier). Deterioration of tissue valves tends to be gradual, and reoperation is rarely an emergency procedure. A patient who needs anticoagulation for chronic atrial fibrillation or prior embolism may as well have a mechanical valve.

Anticoagulation After Surgery

The target International Normalized Ratio with a mechanical valve is 3.0 to 3.5. The addition of low-dose aspirin further lowers the risk of stroke and may be considered for higher risk patients (atrial fibrillation, LA enlargement, history of stroke, or a prosthesis in the mitral position). This combination does carry a higher risk of bleeding (13% had a major bleed during a 4-year follow-up in one study). Many surgeons recommend warfarin for 3 months after placement of a tissue valve and then long-term aspirin.

A common management issue is what to do with anticoagulation when a patient with a mechanical valve needs another surgical procedure. Warfarin must be stopped, and in most cases, it can be restarted soon after surgery. The patient is exposed to a brief period without anticoagulation, and perioperative heparin is not indicated.

When the risk of thromboembolism is especially high, the patient should be admitted 2 days after the last warfarin dose and treated with heparin therapy before and early after surgery. This includes patients with any of the following: an early generation mechanical prostheses (Bjork-Shiley or Starr-Edwards) in the mitral position, double-position prostheses, atrial fibrillation, severe LV dysfunction, a prior embolic event, or a hypercoagulable state.

Medical Therapy for Mitral Regurgitation As afterload is already low, ACE inhibitor therapy probably has little influence on the natural history of the disease. There is no evidence that afterload reduction therapy retards progression of disease in the asymptomatic patient with normal LVEF. On the other hand, symptomatic patients often have low LVEF, and ACE inhibition is indicated for congestive failure whenever LVEF is depressed (you are treating CHF, not the valve). Digoxin may palliate those with depressed LV function, and diuretics are needed to relieve congestion. Those with advanced disease usually have atrial fibrillation and require usual therapy (Chapter 6). As with other valve disease, antibiotic prophylaxis is indicated.

MITRAL VALVE PROLAPSE (MVP) _____

Primary MVP can be inherited or may accompany other connective tissue disorders such as Marfan's syndrome. In such cases other features suggest collagen disorders, including pectus excavatum, straight back, and high arched palate. Secondary MVP may complicate disorders of papillary muscle function or orientation (e.g., ischemic heart disease and cardiomyopathy)

The echocardiographic criteria for MVP have been refined in recent years. Although mild prolapse may be seen in 5% of echocardiograms, the patient with slight posterior motion of the mitral valve leaflets is no longer considered to have the MVP syndrome. Pathologic MVP includes abnormal valve motion plus a thickened, redundant valve, the typical "floppy" or "parachute" valve. The presence of a mid-systolic click on the physical examination is considered diagnostic, even when the echocardiographic findings are unimpressive.

Pathophysiology and Physical Examination

The excursion of the prolapsing valve is increased when the left ventricle is smaller. Thus, the findings of prolapse are magnified by maneuvers that reduce venous return and LV size, such as standing. Amyl nitrate is used for this purpose in the echo laboratory.

The click is mid-systolic, and the murmur follows it. When you hear a late systolic murmur, the most common cause is MVP. Listen carefully for a click, because this finding may be localized to just a small area near the apex or left sternal border.

Diagnosis and Treatment

It is important to avoid overdiagnosis of this condition. Healthy young people often have vague symptoms, including chest pain and palpitations. Do not assign a diagnosis of MVP or "heart disease" when the physical examination is normal and the echo shows mild prolapse and normal valve thickness. Population studies have confirmed that the prognosis is good for those with trivial prolapse, with little risk of stroke or sudden death.

On the other hand, serious complications are possible when there is true MVP (Table 2.3). Interestingly, it is not the thin young woman with mild MVP who is at risk for developing severe MR but the middle-aged man with hypertension. Antibiotic prophylaxis to prevent endocarditis is recommended for those with a systolic murmur or a thickened valve. Mild MVP with no murmur does not require prophylaxis. Aspirin therapy is not indicated for prevention of embolic stroke with mild MVP; although unproved, it is commonly prescribed for severe prolapse.

It is possible but uncommon for severe MVP to cause angina. The "parachute valve" increases papillary muscle tension, creating ischemia. This can lead to an abnormal stress ECG with a perfusion abnormality in the region of the papillary muscle. In such cases, beta blockade may help.

A more common management issue is the patient with mild MVP and vague nonanginal chest pain or palpitations. Monitoring usually shows no arrhythmia during symptoms, and blindly treating either symptom with beta blockade rarely helps. I try not to do stress tests in these young people; false positives are common

TABLE 2.3. Complications of MVP

	Risk	Risk Factors
Infective endocarditis	1% by age 75 No MR: 1/22,000 patients/yr MR: 1/2000 patients/yr	MR, thickened valve (young women with minimal MVP on an echo, no MR, and thin leaflets are at low risk for any complication of MVP)
MR	Men: about 5% by age 75 Women: 1.5% by age 75	Male sex, obesity, hypertension, age > 50
Sudden death	No MR: 2/10,000 MIR: 0.2–1.0%	Severe MR, long QT interval, family history of mitral prolapse with complications
Embolic stroke	Rare; the most recent population studies suggest no risk with mild MVP	Atrial fibrillation, LA enlargement, thickened valve

and add to the confusion. Most now believe that anxiety is responsible for the symptoms. One randomized study showed improvement with a prescribed aerobic exercise program. That seems a sensible approach, because exercise is good for stress management and not bad for the heart. Such symptoms tend to improve with time.

AORTIC STENOSIS

AS is the most common acquired valve lesion. One of my teachers commented that we would all develop AS if we lived 150 years. Exposed to high-velocity flow and considerable turbulence, even a normal aortic valve is bound to stiffen and calcify with time. I tell patients that it is like a carpenter's hand developing callus after years of hammering.

Over an 80-year lifespan, the normal aortic valve does well. On the other hand, if any abnormality of shape increases turbulence, the normal degenerative process is accelerated. The extreme example of this is the bicuspid valve. Stenosis develops in middle age. More commonly, a valve with a minor abnormality, such as a leaflet that is slightly displaced, lasts seven to eight decades before premature calcification and stenosis develop.

It is uncommon for asymptomatic patients with AS to die. Once symptoms develop, the survival curve plunges (Fig. 2.5). Surgical repair is indicated with any one of the classic triad of symptoms: heart failure, angina, or syncope. We like to identify and fix severe AS (a valve area less than 0.75 cm^2) when symptoms

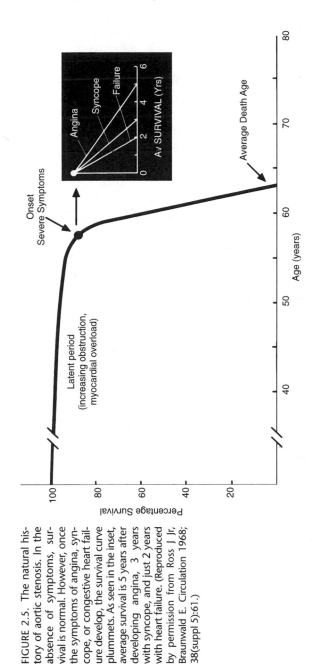

FIGURE 2.5. The natural history of aortic stenosis. In the absence of symptoms, survival is normal. However, once the symptoms of angina, syncope, or congestive heart failure develop, the survival curve plummets. As seen in the inset, average survival is 5 years after developing angina, 3 years with syncope, and just 2 years with heart failure. (Reproduced by permission from Ross J Jr, Braunwald E. Circulation 1968; 38(suppl 5):61.)

are mild, because survival after surgery is related to preoperative status. Those with severe heart failure have a tougher time after surgery.

Pathophysiology, Physical Examination, and Laboratory Evaluation

It is easy to diagnose AS. There is a loud systolic murmur that radiates to the neck. As a consultant I am not asked whether the patient has AS, but whether it is severe. This is another example of simple pathophysiology telling you what to expect on the examination (Fig. 2.6):

1. LV hypertrophy (LVH). The apex impulse is forceful but not displaced. Atrial contraction emptying into a stiff hypertrophied ventricle may cause a palpable glitch or shudder of the upstroke of the apical impulse, the *apical A wave* (Fig. 1.8, my favorite physical finding). The same hemodynamic events produce the S_4 *gallop*, the "stiff ventricle gallop." LVH may be confirmed with the ECG and echocardiogram. *Examination tip:* It helps to roll the patient to the left side to evaluate the quality of the apical impulse and especially to find the apical A wave (it brings the apex closer to your hand). But the position of the apical impulse can only be determined with the patient supine.

2. Evidence for a *calcified valve*. A useful physical sign in elderly patients is the quality of the aortic second sound (A_2). When the valve is heavily calcified, as is usual with senile AS, A_2 softens and then disappears. An *absent A_2* indicates advanced AS. *Examination tip:* How do you tell the difference between the aortic and pulmonic second sounds? Answer: Only A_2 is heard at the right base; P_2 is not loud enough to be heard to the right of the sternum. (An exception to this is marked pulmonary hypertension, uncommon in those with AS.) Thus, absence of S_2 at the right base indicates an absent A_2. Aortic valve calcification may be seen on an overpenetrated chest x-ray and is readily confirmed by echo.

3. Quality and length of the murmur. A mid-systolic, diamond-shaped ejection murmur that ends before S_2 indicates mild AS or aortic valve "sclerosis" rather than stenosis. Severe AS produces a harsh, long murmur that extends almost to S_2 and loses the classic diamond shape. A palpable thrill (the grade 4 murmur) indicates severe stenosis.

4. Delayed LV emptying caused by severe outflow tract obstruction. The physical findings include delay of the arterial

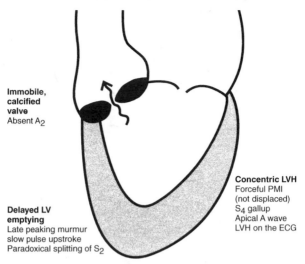

Immobile, calcified valve
Absent A_2

Concentric LVH
Forceful PMI
(not displaced)
S_4 gallup
Apical A wave
LVH on the ECG

Delayed LV emptying
Late peaking murmur
slow pulse upstroke
Paradoxical splitting of S_2

FIGURE 2.6. Pathophysiology of calcific (senile) aortic stenosis and the physical examination. The physical findings that indicate severe AS reflect LVH, delayed LV emptying, and a heavily calcified immobile valve. PMI, point of maximum impulse.

pulse upstroke and paradoxical splitting of S_2. *Examination tip:* Exercise great caution when examining the carotid pulse in elderly patients. There are stories of inexperienced and aggressive examiners provoking stroke. I usually examine the brachial pulse, and gently feel the carotid only if I am uncertain about the pulse contour.

When these physical findings are present, you can count on a high valve gradient (Fig. 2.7) and a valve area below 0.8 cm². Echo-Doppler study confirms the findings, excludes idiopathic hypertrophic subaortic stenosis (IHSS) as an alternative cause of the murmur, and excludes coincidental mitral valve disease.

Timing of Surgery

Cardiac catheterization answers these same questions and with little additional accuracy. A preoperative angiogram is indicated to exclude coronary disease for older patients. AS may cause angina, but about half the patients with AS and angina also have coronary artery disease. Surgery should not be delayed for symptomatic patients with tight AS (valve area less than 0.75 cm²).

For the patient with vague symptoms and borderline hemodynamic findings, what is the danger of a period of observation?

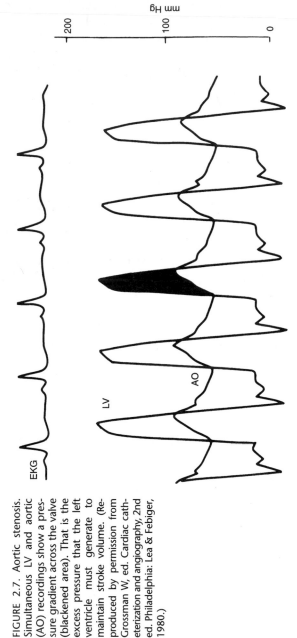

FIGURE 2.7. Aortic stenosis. Simultaneous LV and aortic (AO) recordings show a pressure gradient across the valve (blackened area). That is the excess pressure that the left ventricle must generate to maintain stroke volume. (Reproduced by permission from Grossman W, ed. Cardiac catheterization and angiography, 2nd ed. Philadelphia: Lea & Febiger, 1980.)

Probably not much. In the absence of LV dysfunction at baseline, sudden or irreversible deterioration in contractility is rare. AS is a pressure overload condition. Even when LVEF is depressed with far-advanced, "neglected" disease, it improves after replacing the valve. Uncorking the aorta with valve replacement is the ultimate afterload reduction therapy.

Another concern about delaying surgery is the risk of sudden death with AS. An early British study included a 6-month delay for surgery after cardiac catheterization, and 15% of the patients died while waiting. All of those who died had high LV diastolic pressure and symptomatic heart failure. Sudden death as the first symptom of AS has been described, but it is rare. For those with early disease and no heart failure, observation with repeat echo-Doppler study at 2-year intervals is adequate.

Surgery and Balloon Valvuloplasty (Palliation)

Valve repair is possible in some children with congenital AS. Elderly patients with calcified valves need a prosthesis. Balloon valvuloplasty has been tried as a substitute for surgery for elderly and debilitated patients, and it does reduce the valve gradient and symptoms. The downside is high morbidity and mortality with the procedure and restenosis of the valve within 6 to 12 months. Most centers have given it up.

AORTIC REGURGITATION

AR is caused by diseases of the aortic root (Marfan's syndrome, ankylosing spondylitis, syphilis, or the annuloaortic ectasia of aging) or by conditions affecting the valve leaflets (infective endocarditis, rheumatic fever, congenital bicuspid valve, collagen vascular disease).

Pathophysiology and Physical Examination
Acute AR

This is usually caused by endocarditis, most commonly with staphylococcal infection in a setting of drug abuse. Consider it when there is abrupt onset of heart failure in a young person. Look for peripheral signs of endocarditis (splinter or conjunctival hemorrhages, petechiae), and get blood cultures. A rash could mean gonococcus infection.

The heart murmur may be soft or absent. Acute volume overload of the normal (not dilated) left ventricle causes a marked rise in LV diastolic pressure and severe pulmonary congestion. The stiff pericardium helps to limit LV dilatation. LV diastolic pressure may be similar to aortic diastolic pressure (and arterial pulse pressure is wide). With a small diastolic gradient across the valve, the volume of diastolic regurgitation is minimal, reducing murmur intensity.

Chronic AR

The left ventricle responds to chronic volume overload with eccentric cardiac hypertrophy and dilatation. The enlarged ventricle accommodates the regurgitant volume with little increase in diastolic pressure, so there is no pulmonary congestion. This "chronic compensated" phase of AR may persist for years. Eventually, the left ventricle fails. There is a decline in contractility and a marked increase in LV end-systolic volume without a further increase in stroke volume. LV diastolic pressure rises, leading to pulmonary congestion. Surgery early in this phase of decompensation usually restores normal LV function.

One area of potential confusion is that LVH develops with AR but not with MR, even though both are volume overload conditions. The explanation is that with AR, LV afterload is high. The increased stroke volume with AR all goes to the aorta, leading to an increase in systolic blood pressure and thus an increase in LV afterload (which provokes hypertrophy). With MR, increased LV stroke volume is shared by the aorta and LA, there is no increase in aortic pressure or volume, no rise in afterload, and therefore no LVH (Fig. 2.4).

Interestingly, eccentric hypertrophy with AR is inadequate to normalize wall stress in the dilated left ventricle. Recall Laplace's law:

$$\text{Wall stress or tension} = (\text{pressure} \times \text{radius of the chamber})/\text{wall thickness}$$

Failure of the left ventricle to thicken enough to normalize stress has been called "afterload mismatch." This may cause mild short-term contractile dysfunction, and it contributes to decompensation over the long run.

An important peripheral circulatory response to AR is vasodilatation with low diastolic blood pressure. Pulse pressure is wide. Note that it is wide with acute AR as well, but that is because the valve is essentially wiped out and diastolic LV and arterial pressures are similar. With chronic AR, the valve is still somewhat competent, and there is a considerable difference between LV and aortic diastolic pressure (the "diastolic pressure gradient" between aorta and left ventricle is preserved).

Wide pulse pressure is responsible for a number of physical signs: Corrigan's pulse (sharp upstroke and rapid descent of the carotid pulse), DeMusset's sign (head bobbing), Quincke's pulse (pulsating color in the nail bed with traction on the nail), Hill's sign (augmentation of the systolic pressure in the leg by more than 40 mm Hg compared with the arm), and others. If the pulse pressure is normal, AR probably is not hemodynamically significant.

Treatment

Afterload reduction is a logical treatment for AR; it would at least favor "forward flow." Vasodilatation with nifedipine has been shown to forestall the need for surgery for AR and may be considered for symptomatic patients who will not or cannot have surgery. No data favor afterload reduction prophylactically for asymptomatic patients.

Like other mechanical conditions, a mechanical (surgical) solution is eventually needed. End-systolic LV diameter, an echo measurement, provides the best guide to timing of surgery, much as it does for MR. As long as the left ventricle is able to contract down to a normal volume (end-systolic diameter less than 4.0 cm), it is safe to continue observation. When the end-systolic dimension rises to 5.0 cm, it is time for surgery. Between 4.0 and 5.0 cm, any symptoms would indicate a need for surgery, and periodic echo surveillance is needed for the asymptomatic patient.

An additional indication for surgery is increasing aortic root diameter, a common complication of Marfan's syndrome. When the root diameter exceeds 5.5 to 6.0 cm, the risk of aortic dissection is high, and prophylactic valve plus ascending aorta replacement is needed.

HYPERTROPHIC CARDIOMYOPATHY (HCM) ___

IHSS (idiopathic hypertrophic subaortic stenosis) is a variant of HCM. Hypertrophic cardiomyopathy is a unifying diagnosis of a number of illnesses with common pathophysiology: LVH in the absence of pressure overload. The hypertrophied muscle is histologically abnormal, with disorientation of muscle fibers. Many different terms have been used to describe the condition, and I use IHSS here to focus on outflow tract obstruction.

Aortic outflow tract obstruction is one of four mechanisms that contribute to symptoms in HCM. The others are diastolic dysfunction (see Chapter 1), myocardial ischemia, and arrhythmias.

Pathophysiology and Physical Examination

The subvalvular gradient has been attributed to crowding of the outflow tract by the hypertrophied septum and to movement of the mitral valve leaflet into the outflow tract (Fig. 2.8, Table 2.4). High-velocity flow across this narrowed space creates a Venturi effect, pulling the mitral leaflet into the outflow tract toward the septum, the so-called systolic anterior motion (SAM) of the mitral valve. SAM contributes to obstruction in most patients, and when there is no SAM on the echocardiogram, there is usually no outflow tract gradient. It may be that increased length of the mitral leaflets is not a result of septal hypertrophy but is a primary abnormality of the valve, another feature of the IHSS syndrome.

The outflow tract gradient and murmur increase with lower LV volume. It is a matter of geometry. Less filling of the ventricle means that the outflow tract is narrower, flow velocity and the Venturi effect are heightened, and there is more SAM. Standing after squatting and the strain phase of the Valsalva maneuver lower venous return and accentuate the systolic murmur. In the echo laboratory, amyl nitrite (a venodilator) does the same thing, provoking a gradient, murmur, and SAM.

The systolic murmur is the key diagnostic finding. Unlike valvular AS, there is little radiation of the murmur to the neck (the murmur is generated by MR and outflow tract turbulence). The peripheral pulse also helps differentiate IHSS from valvular AS. With IHSS initial LV emptying is normal, and the pulse

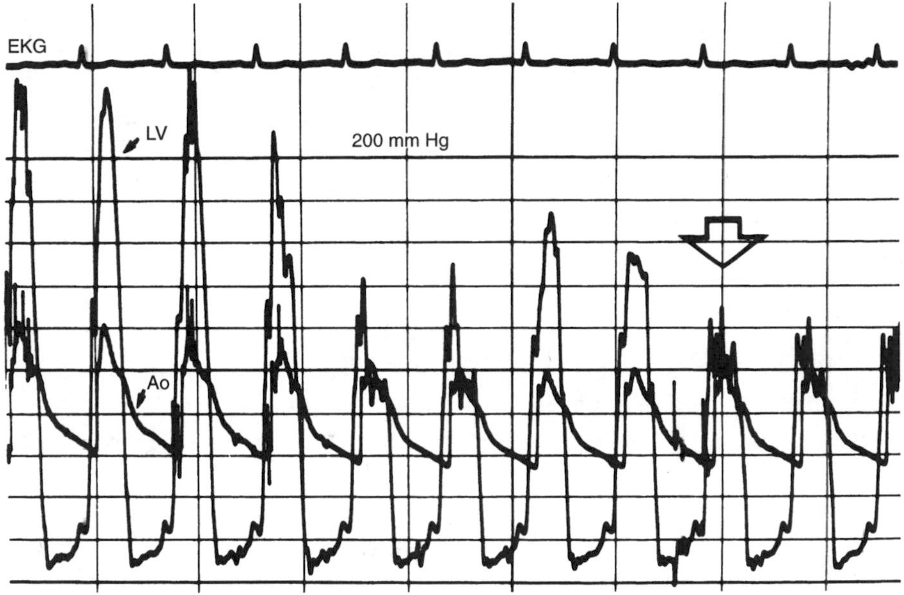

FIGURE 2.8. Hypertrophic cardiomyopathy with left ventricular outflow tract obstruction. These are simultaneous pressures from the left ventricle (LV) and aorta (Ao). Left ventricular pressure is initially measured at the left ventricular apex, the left side of the tracing. As the catheter is withdrawn toward the aortic valve (right side of the tracing), a point is reached just below the valve (arrow) where there is no difference, or gradient, between left ventricular and aortic pressure. This indicates that the level of obstruction is subvalvular, in the body of the ventricle, rather than valvular. (Reproduced by permission from Kern MJ. The cardiac catheterization handbook. St. Louis, MO: Mosby–Year Book, 1991.)

67

TABLE 2.4. Mechanisms of Outflow Tract Obstruction with IHSS

Mechanism	Comment
Hypertrophy of the septum	Unlike most cases of LVH, this is not a response to increased afterload. Instead, there is a lump of histologically abnormal muscle in the septum that crowds the outflow tract (a geometric effect similar to the infundibular stenosis of tetralogy of Fallot). Any intervention that increases LV size also increases the outflow tract dimension (beta blockade, verapamil), and reduction of LV size aggravates obstruction (aggressive diuresis).
Venturi effect	The high-velocity jet across the outflow tract sucks the mitral leaflet toward the LV septum, further aggravating outflow obstruction.
Primary abnormalities of the mitral valve	Increased size and length of leaflets, abnormal orientation of the papillary muscles, and anterior displacement of leaflets have been described. Some believe these changes are inherited as a part of the IHSS syndrome and are not secondary to the Venturi effect.

upstroke is brisk. The stiff left ventricle produces both an S_4 gallop and an apical A wave.

Treatment

Medical treatment of IHSS is directed at increasing space in the outflow tract. Drugs that block contractility (verapamil, beta-blockers, and disopyramide) cause ventricular dilatation, widening the outflow tract and reduced flow velocity, which minimized SAM. The outflow tract gradient is thus relieved. These drugs also improve diastolic function, and other treatment principles for diastolic heart failure apply to IHSS. Maintaining sinus rhythm is critical (see Table 1.8).

Dual-chamber cardiac pacing has also been used. Pacing the right ventricle creates left bundle branch block. Septal activation is thus later in systole, and this septal dyskinesis has been shown to reduce the outflow tract gradient. One randomized trial showed no long-term benefit with pacing, but there are small series that suggest symptomatic benefits.

The newest therapy is "ablation" of septal muscle with local infusion of alcohol through a coronary catheter positioned in the small septal perforating artery. There is immediate reduction of septal contractility and regression of septal hypertrophy over a period of weeks. This technique is replacing surgical myotomy–

myectomy for patients whose symptoms are not adequately controlled with medical therapy.

It should be emphasized that none of the treatments for IHSS have been shown to improve survival. Sudden cardiac death is a possibility and does not appear to be related to the severity of outflow tract obstruction. Sudden death is more likely in younger patients (ages 15 to 35) or when there is extreme LVH, a family history of sudden death, or a history of cardiac arrest or ventricular tachycardia. Nonrandomized studies have suggested a benefit of amiodarone therapy when monitoring shows nonsustained ventricular tachycardia. The implantable defibrillator has been shown to be beneficial.

TRICUSPID REGURGITATION

"The most common cause of right heart failure is left heart failure." Left heart failure is also the most common cause of tricuspid regurgitation (TR). Elevated left atrial and pulmonary venous pressure lead to high pulmonary artery pressure. High right ventricular (RV) pressure and RV dilatation lead to TR. It is especially common for a patient having surgery for mitral valve disease to require tricuspid valve repair. Other causes of pulmonary hypertension, including cor pulmonale and primary pulmonary hypertension, may also cause TR.

Primary TR caused by structural damage to the valve is relatively uncommon. RV infarction, Ebstein's anomaly, endocarditis, and the carcinoid syndrome are illnesses you may encounter on a board examination. Levels of serotonin and its metabolites are higher in those with carcinoid plus tricuspid disease than in others with a normal valve (a flashy tidbit for rounds). Clinically, the most common cause of isolated TR is endocarditis in drug users, termed "right heart endocarditis."

Clinical Presentation, Pathophysiology, and Examination

The typical symptoms are those of right heart failure, including edema, ascites, and fatigue. Hepatic congestion may lead to right upper quadrant pain, especially if the onset is rapid.

The apical impulse is not displaced unless there is LV disease. There is a parasternal lift (recall that the right ventricle is the most anterior cardiac chamber, located just below the sternum and anterior to the left ventricle). P_2 is loud when there is pulmonary hypertension, and this is the one time you may hear both A_2 and P_2 at the right base (normally P_2 is soft and is heard only on the left side). RV gallops may be audible over the sternum and tend to increase with inspiration.

The murmur of TR is holosystolic and best heard along the right sternal border. It increases with inspiration. Negative intrathoracic pressure sucks blood into the chest, increasing RV filling and stroke volume and increasing the TR volume. If there is severe RV failure and stroke volume does not rise with increased filling, the murmur may not change with inspiration.

The jugular venous pressure is elevated, and it is important to examine the jugular venous pulse. Normally, the dominant venous wave is the A wave, generated by atrial systole. But with TR there is no effective valve separating the right ventricle from the jugular vein, so the pressure wave generated by ventricular systole is transmitted back, and the dominant pulsation is the V wave.

Examination tip: The key to examining the jugular vein is to feel the brachial pulse. If the dominant venous pulsation is simultaneous with the arterial pulse, it is a V wave. If the venous pulsation is just before the arterial pulse (presystolic), you are seeing an A wave. With TR, V > A.

The liver is usually enlarged and may be pulsatile, because the V wave is reflected back through the venous circulation.

Treatment

Treatment of TR is usually centered on treating the primary problem (left heart failure, mitral valve disease, or pulmonary hypertension caused by lung disease). When there is no left heart disease, therapy is aimed at relieving symptoms with diuretics. Isolated TR may be tolerated for years, and it is rare that surgical repair is needed.

It is common for TR to complicate mitral valve disease. Frequently, the surgeon fixes the mitral valve, takes the patient off heart–lung bypass, and evaluates the tricuspid valve for persistent regurgitation (traditionally by sticking a finger through a hole in the right atrium and feeling the TR jet). If TR remains severe, the patient goes back on bypass and tricuspid annuloplasty is performed.

BACTERIAL ENDOCARDITIS_____

Pathophysiology

As with most infections, endocarditis requires a susceptible host and exposure to an infecting organism. The major component of susceptibility is a roughened valve or endovascular surface, usually the result of increased turbulence. Fibrin and platelets attach to the roughened surface, and circulating bacteria stick to this thrombus, becoming an independent site of infection able to seed the rest of the body. Valve lesions with a high degree of turbulence are more likely to promote colonization than large defects with high flow but low turbulence (e.g., atrial septal defect).

Almost all bacteria may reach the circulation, but only those able to adhere to thrombus cause endocarditis. For example, *Escherichia coli* and *Klebsiella pneumoniae* usually pass a roughened valve surface and do not stick, even though these are frequent causes of bacteremia in patients with cholangitis or pyelonephritis. On the other hand, *Staphylococcus aureus* is likely to stick to a valve surface in the first circulatory pass and to literally cover the valve within 24 hours.

Clinical Presentation

Fever and other constitutional symptoms such as weight loss, fatigue, and weakness are common with subacute bacterial endocarditis. Virtually every organ in the body may be a target of emboli from the vegetation. Stroke occurs in about one fourth of cases.

On physical examination there is usually a heart murmur. Classic skin lesions include splinter hemorrhages (a picture of nails often appears on board examinations); petechiae involving skin, conjunctiva, or mucous membranes; painful subcutaneous nodules on fingers or toes (Osler's nodes); and painless hemorrhagic macules on the palms and soles (Janeway lesions). Clubbing is common with chronic endocarditis, but it is not specific (think of lung cancer as well). Roth spots are present in only 5% of cases and can also be caused by leukemia, lupus, and profound anemia. Splenomegaly is found in as many as half the cases.

Associated Conditions

Right heart (usually tricuspid valve) endocarditis is commonly associated with intravenous drug abuse. Think of it, as well, for those with indwelling catheters. In urban centers a common cause is methacillin-resistant *S. aureus*, although enterococci, viridans streptococci, and *Pseudomonas aeruginosa* are seen often. These patients are also at risk for candida endocarditis, which may present with endophthalmitis and left-side valvular infection.

More than half the patients with *Streptococcus bovis* endocarditis have lesions in the colon, including malignancies. Other malignancies may predispose to bacteremia and valve infection with unusual organisms such as *Clostridium septicum, Listeria monocytogenes*, and group B β-hemolytic streptococci.

Laboratory Studies

One of the first three blood cultures is positive in more than 95% of cases. When there has been antibiotic treatment in the previous 2 weeks, the yield falls to 65%. For the initial evaluation of the untreated patient, three sets of cultures are adequate. A patient who has had antibiotic therapy should have blood cultures 2 and 10 days after treatment ends.

Constitutional symptoms are usually accompanied by elevated sedimentation rate or positive rheumatoid factor, but negative studies do not exclude endocarditis. In Petersdorf's classic study, the mean Westergren sedimentation rate was 57 mm/hr. Normocytic anemia is present in most cases, and it worsens with time. The white cell count is elevated only occasionally.

The echocardiogram demonstrates valvular vegetations and is now included in diagnostic criteria for endocarditis. Small vegetations may be detected with transesophageal study. But the echo may have both false-positive and false-negative results. The test is more sensitive than specific. Note that vegetations may persist for 2 years or longer after successful treatment, so a vegetation on the valve does not prove active infection. Other imaging studies usually do not help; gallium scans have been used, but the results are unimpressive.

Acute Bacterial Endocarditis

Rapid destruction of a valve is possible, most commonly with staphylococcal or gonococcal sepsis. Acute AR (or, less commonly,

MR) leads to severe pulmonary congestion or shock. As noted, the regurgitant murmur may be soft or absent.

Endocarditis is suggested by the abrupt onset of heart failure. Other clinical evidence for infection may include fever, the rash of gonococcemia, and elevated white count. A history of drug abuse is common when the patient is young and has no prior history of heart disease. As with subacute endocarditis, there may be evidence for peripheral embolus.

Treatment

Since the days of Osler, the incidence of viridans streptococcal endocarditis has fallen from almost 100% of the cases to less than 25%. Other frequent causes of endocarditis, such as enterococcus and staphylococcus, are less susceptible to antibiotic therapy and much trickier to manage. Frankly, few cardiologists are qualified to do it. We quickly turn to our infectious disease colleagues for the choice of antibiotics and appropriate monitoring. (This is, of course, the *cardiology* rotation.)

Patients who are acutely ill may require empiric therapy, before culture results are available. Start a combination of nafcillin or vancomycin plus an aminoglycoside.

A common issue for the cardiology consultant is whether to recommend surgery. The classic indications for valve replacement are heart failure, major emboli, and persistent bacteremia. In recent years there has been a trend toward earlier replacement of infected valves. For example, a patient with an increasing diuretic requirement may benefit from surgery. Difficult to treat organisms are relative indications for early surgery, including *P. aeruginosa* or fungi, especially when fever resolves slowly with antibiotic therapy. In many centers, surgery is becoming standard treatment for staphylococcal endocarditis (believing it better to operate early, before perivalvular abscesses develop).

Prosthetic valve infection usually requires surgery. An exception is endocarditis more than 2 months after surgery with an especially susceptible organism such as viridans streptococci. Any dysfunction of the prosthetic valve, especially perivalvular leak, indicates a need for surgery (listen carefully for the murmur of AR).

When there is an indication for surgery, the patient with both native and prosthetic valve endocarditis has a better chance if the operation is not delayed. With time, there is greater opportunity

TABLE 2.5. **Risk of Infective Endocarditis**

Endocarditis prophylaxis recommended
  Highest risk
    Prosthetic cardiac valves
    Previous endocarditis
    Complex cyanotic congenital heart disease
  Moderate risk
    Most other congenital cardiac conditions (with the following exceptions)
    Acquired valvular dysfunction
    IHSS
    MVP with regurgitation or thickened leaflets
Endocarditis prophylaxis not recommended (low risk)
    Isolated secundum atrial septal defect
    After surgical repair of atrial septal defect or patent ductus arteriosus (without
      residua after 6 mo)
    After coronary artery bypass surgery
    MVP without regurgitation or thickened leaflets
    Physiologic or functional heart murmur (no valve abnormality on echo)
    Previous rheumatic fever without valve abnormality
    Cardiac pacemaker and implanted defibrillators

for the organism to burrow into the myocardium, cause abscesses (heart block is a potential consequence—watch the PR interval), and generate emboli. Even though the new valve is placed into an area that may not be completely sterile, it is rare that the original organism infects it.

The replacement valve may not sit as securely into the valve ring because of weakened tissue. Significant perivalvular leak complicates about 15% of operations for active endocarditis. Antibiotic therapy after surgery is a complex issue requiring infectious disease consultation.

Prevention of Endocarditis

Most valvular disease is an indication for antibiotic prophylaxis (Table 2.5). Patients with MVP but no murmur rarely develop endocarditis. Either a murmur or Doppler evidence for substantial MR is an indication for antibiotic prophylaxis. Men over 45 years old with MVP, even without a murmur, should have antibiotic prophylaxis because this group is at highest risk for endocarditis.

Invasive dental, gastrointestinal, genitourinary, and upper respiratory tract procedures are indications for prophylaxis. On the other hand, restorative dentistry (filling teeth), endotracheal intubation, esophageal endoscopy, and vaginal delivery are not, except for highest risk patients. Cardiac catheterization does not require prophylaxis. Antibiotic prophylaxis regimens are updated periodically by the American Heart Association and are found in most standard texts (the dentist usually has this information).

SUGGESTED READINGS _____

Mitral Valve Disease

Harris KM, Robiolio P. Valvular heart disease. Identifying and managing mitral and aortic lesions. Postgrad Med 1999;106:113–125.

Horstkotte D, Schulte HD, Niehues R, et al. Diagnostic and therapeutic considerations in acute, severe mitral regurgitation: experience in 42 consecutive patients entering the intensive care unit with pulmonary edema. J Heart Valve Dis 1993;2:512–520.

Lax D, Eicher M, Goldbeg SJ. Mild dehydration induces echocardiographic signs of mitral valve prolapse in healthy females with prior normal cardiac findings. Am Heart J 1992;124:1533–1540. (Anything that reduces LV size [dehydration, upright posture, nitrates] may provoke mild prolapse. It also accentuates the physical findings of prolapse.)

Mazur T, Parilak KD, Kaluza G, et al. Balloon valvuloplasty for mitral stenosis. Curr Opin Cardiol 1999;14:95–103. (A thorough review.)

Nishimura RA, McGoon MD. Perspectives on mitral valve prolapse. N Engl J Med 1999;341:48–50. (An editorial that clears the air about diagnostic criteria for the MVP syndrome. Only patients with billowing, thickened, myxomatous valves appear at risk for the late complications of MVP. Using stricter diagnostic criteria, two other articles in this issue of the journal indicate a relatively low incidence [2.4%] of MVP in a community population [page 1 of the July 1 issue] and an absence of any connection between MVP and stroke in young patients [page 8].)

Reardon MJ, David TE. Mitral valve replacement with preservation of the subvalvular apparatus. Curr Opin Cardiol 1999;14:104–110. (A good review of the history of mitral valve surgery, and a description of surgical techniques.)

Reusser L, Crawford MH. Timing of mitral valve replacement surgery. Prim Cardiol 1993;19:15–21.

Roy SB, Gopinath N. Mitral stenosis. Circulation 1968;38(suppl 2):68–79. (It is interesting that the best general reviews of rheumatic heart disease are this old.)

Rozich JD, Carabello BA, Usher BW, et al. Mitral valve replacement with and without chordal preservation in patients with chronic mitral regurgitation: mechanism for differences in postoperative ejection performance. Circulation 1992;86:1718–1724.

Scordo KA. Effects of aerobic exercise training on symptomatic women with mitral valve prolapse. Am J Cardiol 1991;67:863–868.

Turi ZG, Reyes VP, Raju BS, et al. Percutaneous balloon versus surgical closed commissurotomy for mitral stenosis: a prospective, randomized trial. Circulation 1991;83:1179–1185.

Tuzcu EM, Block PC, Friffin BP, et al. Immediate and long-term outcome of percutaneous mitral valvotomy in patients 65 years and older. Circulation 1992;85:963–971. (Age is not a contraindication, but the procedure works best when there is little calcification or mitral regurgitation. Severe calcification is common in elderly patients with MS.)

Waller BF, Howard J, Fess S. Pathology of mitral valve stenosis and pure mitral regurgitation. II. Clin Cardiol 1994;17:395–402.

Ward C, Hancock BW. Extreme pulmonary hypertension caused by mitral valve disease: natural history and results of surgery. Br Heart J 1975;2:574–82. (It is possible to have right heart failure and high pulmonary artery pressure "behind" high left atrial pressure and mitral stenosis. Unlike Eisenmenger's syndrome, the pulmonary hypertension is not fixed and usually resolves after surgery.)

Wisenbaugh T, Spann JF, Carabello BA. Differences in myocardial performance and load between patients with similar amounts of chronic aortic versus chronic mitral regurgitation. J Am Coll Cardiol 1984;3:916–22.

Aortic Valve Disease

Bonow RO, Lakatos E, Maron JB, Epstein SE. Serial long-term assessment of the natural history of asymptomatic patients with chronic aortic regurgitation and normal left ventricular systolic function. Circulation 1991;84:1625–1630.

Carabello, BA. Timing of valve replacement in aortic stenosis. Circulation 1997;95:2241–2242.

Lindroos M, Kupari M, Heikkila J. Aortic valve abnormalities in old age: common and operable. Cardiol Board Rev 1994;11: 43–55.

Matthews AW, Barritt DW, Keen GE, Belsey RH. Preoperative mortality in aortic stenosis. Br Heart J 1974;36:101–103. (Fascinating report of patients who waited 6 months for surgery, after cardiac catheterization. The 15% who died were severely symptomatic. Sudden death is rarely the first symptom of AS.)

Otto CM, Lind BK, Ktizman DW, et al. Association of aortic valve sclerosis with cardiovascular mortality and morbidity in the elderly. N Engl J Med 1999;341:142–146. (A thickened aortic valve with minimal outflow tract obstruction is a common finding among elderly patients, about 30% in this study. The risk of progression to significant stenosis is low, about 8% per year. However, this large population study found an increased risk of myocardial infarction and cardiovascular death with aortic sclerosis, probably because it is a marker for underlying coronary artery disease [see the editorial in the same issue by Carabello].)

Pellikka PA, Nishimura RA, Bailey KR,Tajik AJ. The natural history of adults with symptomatic, hemodynamically significant aortic stenosis. J Am Coll Cardiol 1990;15:1012–1019.

Roger VL, Tajik AJ, Bailey KR, et al. Progression of aortic stenosis in adults: new appraisal using Doppler echocardiography. Am Heart J 1990;86:1718–1726.

Rosenhek R, Binder T, Porenta G, et al. Predictors of outcome in severe, asymptomatic aortic stenosis. N Engl J Med 2000; 343:611–617. (It is usually safe to delay surgery until symptoms develop. Heavy valve calcification and a rapid change in the aortic-jet velocity on serial echos indicate poor prognosis and would favor earlier surgery.)

Scognamiglio R, Rahimtoola SH, Fasoli G, et al. Nifedipine in asymptomatic patients with severe aortic regurgitation and normal left ventricular function. N Engl J Med 1994;331:689–693. (Vasodilator therapy improves hemodynamics and can forestall the need for surgery.)

Hypertrophic Cardiomyopathy

Corrado D, Basso C, Schiavon M. Screening for hypertrophic cardiomyopathy in young athletes. N Engl J Med 1998;339: 364–369.

Kurowski K, Chandran S. The preparticipation athletic evaluation. Am Fam Physician 2000;61:2683–2698. (Echocardiography is not indicated unless the patient has a family history of hypertrophic cardiomyopathy or sudden death or there is an abnormal physical examination [have the patient Valsalva when screening for the murmur of IHSS].)

Maron BJ. Role of alcohol septal ablation in treatment of obstructive hypertrophic cardiomyopathy. Lancet 2000;355:425–426. (This is the way we are treating hypertrophic cardiomyopathy presently. Symptoms improve with a lower outflow tract gradient. How this will affect the natural history of the illness is uncertain at this time.)

Maron BJ, Nishimura RA, McKenna WJ, et al. Assessment of permanent dual-chamber pacing as a treatment for drug-refractory symptomatic patients with obstructive hypertrophic cardiomyopathy;

a randomized, double-blind, crossover study. Circulation 1999;99:2927–2933.

Sprito P, Bellone P, Harris KM, et al. Magnitude of left ventricular hypertrophy and risk of sudden death in hypertrophic cardiomyopathy. N Engl J Med 2000;342:1778–1785. (A review of records from 480 patients. Asymptomatic patients with extreme LVH [wall thickness ≥ 30 mm] had a 40% risk of sudden death. Most of the highest risk patients were young and had few or no other symptoms. Patients with wall thickness ≤ 19 mm had close to zero risk. Other predictors of sudden death with IHSS are a family history for sudden death [in two or more young family members] or a history of prior cardiac arrest or symptomatic ventricular tachycardia. Amiodarone has been suggested for prevention of sudden death based upon retrospective studies, but these authors suggest implantable defibrillator therapy.)

Sprito P, Seidman CE, McKenna WJ, Maron BJ. The management of hypertrophic cardiomyopathy. N Engl J Med 1997;336:775–785. (Excellent review.)

Infective Endocarditis

Giessel BE, Koenig CJ, Blake RL Jr. Management of bacterial endocarditis. Am Fam Physician 2000;61:1725–1739.

Osmon DR. Antimicrobial prophylaxis in adults. Mayo Clin Proc 2000;75:98–109.

CHAPTER 3

Atherosclerosis and Lipid Disorders

The number of cardiac deaths in the United States has been relatively constant at 750,000 per year in the last decade, and coronary artery disease (CAD) is responsible for 60% of them. CAD is a disease of both middle and old age; 45% of myocardial infarctions occur in people less than 65 years old. The economic burden is huge; in 1996, the estimated direct cost of cardiovascular disease in the United States was $259 billion.

There is a misconception that CAD is predominantly a man's disease. Although women tend to develop it a decade later, they have a similar risk of death from CAD. It is the leading cause of death for women and men. As a rule, all ethnic groups that share a diet rich in animal fats are at risk.

ATHEROSCLEROSIS

Response-to-Injury Hypothesis of Atherogenesis

The intimal surface of arteries is lined with endothelial cells that form a barrier between elements of the blood and the arterial wall. The first step in atherogenesis appears to be endothelial injury and increased permeability of this barrier. The nature of early vascular injury is uncertain, and multiple factors may interact. There is increased shear stress and turbulence at branch points, a common site of plaque development. Infection has been proposed, because both viral elements and chlamydia have been isolated from plaque (though their presence does not prove causality). Oxidized low-density-lipoprotein (LDL) cholesterol is cytotoxic and appears to have a major role in endothelial injury.

After disruption of the endothelial barrier, the next step is the complex interaction of a number of different cell types, which

79

TABLE 3.1. Cellular Elements that Contribute to Atherosclerotic Plaque Formation

Cell Type	Actions
Endothelial cells	The first step in atherogenesis is endothelial injury with cell–cell separation. Subsequent endothelial dysfunction includes inappropriate vasoconstriction or vasodilation, production of growth factors, procoagulant activity, and loss of the permeability buffer.
Monocytes/ macrophages	Monocytes are attracted to the injured endothelium, penetrate to subendothelial regions, and are transformed to macrophages. These secrete growth factors, mitogens for smooth muscle cells, and factors promoting migration of both smooth muscle cells and fibroblasts. They also secrete oxidized LDL and/or superoxide anion that further injure endothelium and other cells in the developing plaque.
Platelets	Platelets are attracted to injured endothelium, adhere, and aggregate. The platelet thrombus releases growth factors (as do the other cell types).
Smooth muscle cells	In response to growth factors, they migrate from the media into the intima and then proliferate. They may be transformed to foam cells. In cell culture, smooth muscle cells are able to produce growth factors and connective tissue.

leads to propagation of endothelial injury and infiltration of lipids and other blood elements into deeper layers of the arterial wall (Table 3.1). Circulating, oxidized LDL binds to monocytes and facilitates their migration into the endothelium where they become macrophages. These cells scavenge more lipid, particularly oxidized LDL, become foam cells, and form the "fatty streak." Activated macrophages produce cytotoxic substances that promote further endothelial injury. They also produce growth factors that stimulate proliferation and migration of smooth muscle cells into the early plaque. In turn, smooth muscle cells secrete growth factors and cytokines and produce connective tissue. As the plaque matures, the fibroproliferative process dominates with replication of smooth muscle cells, attraction of fibroblasts, and production of connective tissue. The core of the mature plaque is rich in lipid.

Platelets have an important role. They adhere to injured endothelium, particularly at branch points where there is turbulence and stasis. Like other cellular elements, they produce growth factors and vasoactive substances. Platelets are critical to the genesis of unstable syndromes. Advanced lesions commonly develop surface cracks and fissures. Platelets immediately adhere to exposed collagen on the injured plaque and form mural thrombi that may be organized and incorporated into the plaque; this is the probable mechanism of rapid disease progression and unstable angina. Arterial occlusion by mural thrombus is the usual mechanism for myocardial infarction. Clinical trials have shown that blocking platelet function is far more effective than other forms of anticoagulation for the prevention of these unstable coronary syndromes.

Angiotensin II also works at the endothelial level. It promotes endothelial dysfunction as a vasoconstrictor, and it is involved in the genesis of superoxide radical by macrophages (promoting uptake of oxidized LDL by the macrophage). Tissue active ACE inhibitors are being studied as therapy to prevent atherosclerosis and unstable coronary syndromes.

Risk Factors

The Framingham Study reported its 6-year follow-up in 1961 and established the concept of risk factors for premature atherosclerosis. A risk factor identifies individuals with a greater chance of developing disease, and it *may be* a cause of the disease. But causality is only proven when a clinical trial shows that correction of the risk factor prevents disease ("primary prevention") or halts the progression of already established disease ("secondary prevention"). Known and suspected risk factors for atherosclerosis are summarized in Table 3.2.

Even without proof of causality, risk factor modification is the cornerstone for treatment of all atherosclerotic conditions. There is no uncertainty about the treatment of major risk factors. Braunwald reviewed more recently described—and less certain—risk factors (Table 3.2) and suggested that standard therapy in the future could include folate (to reduce homocysteine levels), niacin (to lower fibrinogen, LDL cholesterol, and lipoprotein(a) [Lp(a)] levels and to raise high-density-lipoprotein [HDL] cholesterol), aspirin (specifically to reduce the risk of myocardial infarction in those with elevated C-reactive protein), and antibiotic therapy for those with chlamydial infection. Watch for these in future clinical trials.

A particularly difficult risk factor to treat is cigarette smoking, and the current approach is outlined in Table 3.3. Using it,

TABLE 3.2. Risk Factors for Atherosclerotic Cardiovascular Disease (ASCVD)

Risk Factor	Current Evidence (there are many studies, and the following is not inclusive but instead provides examples of available data)
Dyslipidemia	Lowering cholesterol by 1% reduces the incidence of CAD by 2%. Raising HDL also reduces the incidence of CAD. Treatment of hyperlipidemia reduces mortality and morbidity.
Hypertension	SHEP showed that control of systolic pressure lowers the risk of 1) fatal and nonfatal stroke, 2) nonfatal myocardial infarction (MI) plus coronary death, 3) combined ASCVD outcomes. A meta-analysis of 14 trials showed that lowering blood pressure 6 mm Hg reduced the CAD event rate 14%.
Diabetes mellitus	A risk factor for all, but with a greater effect on women. In addition to increasing ASCVD, it also increases the risk of heart failure. Diabetes also indicates a worse prognosis for those with ASCVD. Clinical trials support treating diabetic patients as though they already have ASCVD, lowering LDL to < 100 mg/dL.
Cigarette smoking	There is a "dose–response" curve: the number of cigarettes per day is proportional to the incidence of multiple ASCVD end points (CAD, stroke, PVD, and death).
Family history	After stratifying for other risk factors, a positive family history increased risk 2–4-fold for various ASCVD end points.
Male sex	Premature disease is more common in men. (Nevertheless, CAD is the leading cause of death in women, with the onset about 10 years later.)
Age	About four fifths of fatal MI occur in those ≥65 years old.
Obesity	Abdominal and truncal obesity is related to insulin resistance, hyperlipidemia, and hypertension (a constellation referred to as "syndrome X"). The Framingham study identified obesity as an independent predictor of ASCVD.

table continues

you may expect sustained (6 months) abstinence in 20% to 40% of patients, depending on the effectiveness of behavioral therapy.

LIPIDS

A number of clinical trials have proven that elevated cholesterol causes vascular disease (Table 3.4). You will not need this much detail for board examinations, but you may find the information useful when on rounds. It is important to understand the difference between "primary" and "secondary" prevention. Stopping the progression of disease in a patient who already has it (secondary prevention) justifies more aggressive treatment than preventing disease in one who does not have it (primary prevention).

TABLE 3.2. *(continued)*

Risk Factor	Current Evidence (there are many studies, and the following is not inclusive but instead provides examples of available data)
Left ventricular hypertrophy	An independent predictor of CAD, particularly for older people. Also indicates poor prognosis for those with CAD.
Physical inactivity	In the MRFIT study those who exercised had a 27% lower CAD mortality rate.
Stress, mood, and personality type	Proposed risk factors include "negative affectivity," social inhibition, and type A personality. The evidence is mixed. Anger is associated with onset of MI, and both MI and sudden death are more common on Monday morning. Depression predicts a poor outcome after MI. We have been referring patients to our mind–body clinic that teaches meditation techniques, etc. Evidence for efficacy is soft; two randomized trials failed to show survival benefits of nonspecific interventions for general distress after MI.
Homocysteine	Related to deficiency of vitamins B_6 and B_{12} and folic acid. About 20–30% of patients with ASCVD have elevated homocysteine, compared with 2% in control populations. It may be as important as hypercholesterolemia, and it is easily treated with vitamins (a developing story in the treatment of ASCVD).
Hemostatic factors	Fibrinogen, coagulation factor VII, and plasminogen activator inhibitor 1 have all been reported to be elevated in patients with CAD, as has reduced fibrinolytic activity.
Inflammation	Elevated C-reactive protein indicates increased risk for acute coronary syndromes.
Chlamydia pneumoniae	Infection is possibly related to atherogenesis and plaque instability. Bacteria have been isolated from plaque.

PVD, peripheral vascular disease; MRFIT, multiple risk factor intervention trial (see Table 3.4).

Current treatment recommendations by the National Cholesterol Education Program (NCEP) are listed in Table 3.5.

Lipoprotein Metabolism

Oil and water do not mix. Cholesterol and triglycerides are hydrophobic, like oil, and do not mix in blood (which is aqueous). To get fats to dissolve in water requires a chemical that works like soap or detergent: a molecule that binds to fat on one side and to water on the other.

The lipoprotein particle has a core of fat packaged with a specialized protein that works like a detergent. This protein molecule, called an apoprotein, has regions that are nonpolar (hydrophobic) that bind with lipids and other regions that are

TABLE 3.3. An Approach to Smoking Cessation

Behavioral modification	Works at multiple levels: 1) The practitioner should mention tobacco at every visit (one survey reported that 50% of doctors failed to comment on continued smoking). 2) Smoking cessation clinic: this intense approach focuses on skills building (teaches the patient how to resist smoking, to use substitute behaviors, to make the home-car-office smoke free, to avoid alcohol while stopping). 3) Social support: enlist family, friends, and the medical team to help with positive reinforcement (threatening a bad outcome is less successful).
Nicotine replacement	Patients usually have a preference for gum, nasal spray, or patch. Consider starting with a "kit" containing all three, and encourage the patient to experiment (although staying within the recommended dose range). Start replacement the day of the last cigarette. I usually suggest no reduction in the nicotine dose until the new behavior (nonsmoking) is well entrenched. Advise the patient not to smoke while on replacement therapy.
Antidepressant therapy	Smoking has an antidepressant effect, and there is mild "rebound" depression with cessation that is blocked by bupropion. Rx: sustained release bupropion (Zyban or Wellbutrin) 150 mg twice daily. (Start with 150 mg once daily for 3 days, then increase the dose.) Start it a week before the patient stops smoking, as 1 week is needed to reach a steady-state blood level. Have the patient set a date to stop smoking. Continue therapy for 7–12 weeks. If still smoking at 7 weeks, this will not be a successful quit attempt, and you may as well stop the drug.

polar (hydrophilic) that face the surrounding aqueous phase and form hydrogen bonds with water. The lipid–apoprotein package is thus water soluble.

An additional property of apoproteins is binding sites that regulate steps in lipid metabolism. For example, the apoB-100 protein on the surface of the LDL cholesterol particle is recognized by the liver's LDL receptor, allowing hepatic uptake of LDL. Other apoproteins are cofactors for enzymes that interact with lipoproteins, such as lipoprotein lipase.

The core of fat in the lipoprotein particle includes fatty acids, cholesterol esters, phospholipid, and triglycerides. Lipoproteins vary in density, and the first measurement techniques and classifications schemes used ultracentrifugation. Larger, less-dense particles contain more triglyceride and do not migrate as far in the centrifuge. Thus, very-low-density lipoprotein (VLDL), which is fluffy stuff with 55% triglyceride, 19% cholesterol, and only 8% protein, migrates the least. The highest density lipopro-

TABLE 3.4. Clinical Trials of Lipid Altering Therapy

Study	Drug	Number of Patients/Follow-up	Results
Primary Prevention Trials			
Lipid Research Clinics–Coronary Primary Prevention Trial (LRC-CPPT)	Cholestyramine 24 g/d	3806 men, 35–39 yr old; 7 years	Total cholesterol down 8.5%, LDL down 12.6%. CAD mortality and morbidity (nonfatal MI) reduced 19%. No change in all-cause mortality.
Helsinki Heart Trial	Gemfibrozil 1200 mg/d	4801 men, 40–55 yr old; 5 years	LDL down 11%, HDL up 11 %. Cardiac events (death or MI) down 34%; nonfatal MI down 37%. No effect on all-cause mortality. This trial established low HDL as an independent risk factor.
Multiple Risk Factor Intervention Trial (MRFIT)	Diet plus other risk factors modified	12,866 men, 35–57 yr old; >10 years	10.5-year cardiovascular mortality down 7.9%; 24% fewer deaths from MI.
West of Scotland Primary Prevention Trial	Pravastatin vs. placebo	>6000 men; 5 years	LDL down 26%. Death from CAD down 28%, nonfatal MI down 31%.
Secondary Prevention Trials			
Coronary Drug Project (CDP)	5 drugs tested; niacin 3 g/d most effective	8341 men after MI, 30–64 yr old; 15 years	Niacin: total cholesterol down 10%. All-cause mortality down 11%, primarily due to lowered CAD mortality.
Scandinavian Simvastatin Survival Study (4S)	Simvastatin vs. placebo	4444 men and women with stable CAD, 35–77 y, old; 5.5 y	LDL down 38%. All cause mortality down 30%, and coronary events down 40%. Strokes down 30%.
Angiographic Trials *(there have been many, and these are representative)*			
Familial Atherosclerosis Study (FATS)	Colestipol (a resin) alone vs. colestipol plus niacin or lovastatin	men ≤ 62 yr old with known CAD. Recath after 2.5 yr	Progression of disease in 46% on colestipol alone ("controls") vs. 21% and 25% with lovastatin or niacin. Regression of plaque in 11% of controls vs. 32% and 39% with lovastatin or niacin. Death or MI in 19% controls vs. 6% and 4% with lovastatin or niacin.
Cholesterol Lowering Atherosclerosis Study (CLAS)	Colestipol 30 g/d + niacin 3–12 g/d	188 men after bypass surgery; 2- and 4-yr follow-up	Total cholesterol down 27%, LDL down 43%, HDL up 37%. Less progression of CAD, and 16% had plaque regression. 4-yr follow-up showed even better results.

MI, myocardial infarction.

TABLE 3.5. National Cholesterol Education Program Guidelines:
An Emphasis on LDL Cholesterol

Patient Profile	Initiate Drug Therapy if the LDL Cholesterol Is:	Target LDL Cholesterol
<2 other CAD risk factors, and no active CAD	≥190 mg/dL after 6 mo of diet therapy	<160 mg/dL
≥2 other risk factors and no CAD	≥160 mg/dL after 6 mo of diet therapy	<130 mg/dL
Known CAD or other atheroslcerotic disease[a]	≥130 mg/dL after 6–12 wk of diet therapy	<100 mg/dl

[a]Based on recent clinical trials, most clinicians start reductase therapy for any patient with established disease and LDL cholesterol above 100 mg/dL and without the trial of diet therapy. In addition, other studies support a target level of LDL, 80 mg/dL. Whether "lower is better" is the subject of ongoing clinical trials.

tein (HDL) by weight has just 5% triglycerides and a higher proportion of protein (40%) and cholesterol (22%) and migrates the farthest in the centrifuge. Between the two is the LDL particle, which has the largest percentage of cholesterol (50%), 6% triglyceride, and 22% protein.

The apoproteins on the surface of the lipoprotein particles can now be measured using antibody techniques; apoA is found on HDL and apoB-100 primarily on LDL. Thus, a patient with a high apoB level will also have an elevated LDL level. It helps to know what your clinical laboratory is doing. Most common is the centrifugation technique that isolates the entire lipoprotein molecule (fat core plus the apoprotein envelope) and then measures just the lipid component. Thus, when the laboratory reports the LDL cholesterol level, it is understood that the LDL component has been isolated from the other lipoproteins by centrifugation, the apoprotein envelope separated from the lipid core, and the cholesterol contained in the lipid core measured and reported as mg cholesterol/dL. This is what you usually get from the clinical laboratory, although you will encounter research studies that refer to apoprotein levels.

Metabolic Pathways

A concept that is key to understanding lipoprotein metabolism is that plasma lipoprotein particles are constantly being remodeled. Under the influence of several enzymes, core lipids and apoprotein can be transferred from or among particles, altering their density (and therefore the class). Some of these particle-altering reactions occur in the liver, others in circulating plasma, and others in peripheral tissue.

Exogenous fat transport, or the movement of fat from the intestinal lumen, involves processes different from those that handle stored fat (*endogenous transport*). Here is a "big picture" description of the two transport systems: Both begin by packaging lipid, predominantly triglyceride but some cholesterol as well, into a large particle. This is subjected to a series of lipolytic reactions, with hydrolysis of triglyceride to fatty acids that melt away from the particle. The remodeled particle is smaller and more dense, contains less triglyceride, and therefore has proportionately more cholesterol. Small particles are cleared from the circulation by the liver through the action of specialized receptors on the hepatic cell membrane.

Genetic derangement of a specific step in these metabolic pathways causes "dyslipidemia" and explains why CAD runs in families (Table 3.6). When reviewing the pathways (below), also follow Table 3.6 to better understand the genetics of hyperlipidemia.

Exogenous Fat Transport

Figure 3.1 illustrates exogenous fat transport. Dietary fats are absorbed by the intestinal epithelial cell. Once in the cell the cholesterol is esterified into long-chain fatty acids. Apoproteins are added, and the particle is secreted as a *chylomicron.* Most of the fat in the chylomicron is triglyceride. Lipoprotein lipase located in vascular endothelial cells—especially in muscle and adipose tissue capillary beds—hydrolyzes the triglyceride to free fatty acid, either for storage or as a source of energy. What is left is the *chylomicron remnant*, which is cleared by liver cells.

This process of transporting dietary fat is fairly rapid. Thus, the lipid profile measured after 12 hours of fasting does not reflect exogenous fat transport.

Endogenous Fat Transport

Figure 3.2 illustrates endogenous fat transport. A 70-kg person has roughly 10 kg of triglyceride stored in adipose tissue. Lipases, inhibited by insulin and stimulated by epinephrine, hydrolyze stored triglyceride and release free fatty acid from adipose tissue

TABLE 3.6. Genetic Dyslipidemias

Syndrome	Mechanism	Clinical features
Disorders of Triglycerides		
Familial combined dyslipidemia (high triglycerides and LDL, low HDL)	Overproduction of apoB-100 leading to an excess of VLDL particles. The LDL particles are small and dense (and are thought more atherogenic). The apoB-100 to serum LDL ratio is >1.	Common, and it causes CAD. There is usually a family history of CAD and high triglycerides. Exam: corneal arcus, tuberoeruptive xanthoma (when triglycerides are very high).
Chylomicronemia	Deficiency in lipoprotein lipase or an abnormal apoC-II (needed to activate lipoprotein lipase)	Rare. There is no increase in the risk of vascular disease. Exam: tuberoeruptive xanthoma and xanthelasma.
Familial hypertriglyceridemia	The liver produces large fluffy VLDL particles. The apoB-100 level is normal (the ratio of apoB-100 to LDL is ≤1).	Little increase in the risk of vascular disease. Tuberoeruptive xanthoma. With marked elevation of triglycerides there is a risk of pancreatitis.
Type III dyslipidemia	Combination of familial combined dyslipidemia plus abnormal apoE apoprotein (Fig. 3.1), which binds to the chylomicron remnant receptor. There is accumulation of IDL, which has equal quantities of triglycerides and cholesterol (the levels of the two are thus similar).	Rare. There is a higher incidence of CAD. Exam: orange palmar creases (deposits of IDL). They are quite sensitive to diet therapy.
LDL Disorders		
Familial hypercholesterolemia (high LDL, normal HDL and triglycerides)	Abnormal, ineffective LDL receptor. Heterozygous carriers have about 50% ineffective receptors. The rare homozygote dies in the second decade of life.	Autosomal dominant. Incidence of heterozygous state is 1 in 500. CAD is common, especially in female smokers. Exam: arcus and tendonous xanthoma.
Familial defective apoB-100	The defective apoprotein fails to bind to the LDL receptor.	Uncommon. The clinical syndrome and laboratory findings are similar to familial hypercholesterolemia.

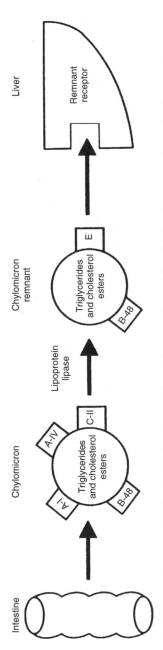

FIGURE 3.1. Exogenous fat transport. A-I, A-IV, B-48, C-II, and E are apolipoproteins. C-II functions as a cofactor for the enzyme, lipoprotein lipase, and E interacts with the "remnant receptor" on the hepatocyte. (Reproduced by permission from Breslow JL. Lipoprotein metabolism. Cardiol Board Rev 1989;6:10–15.)

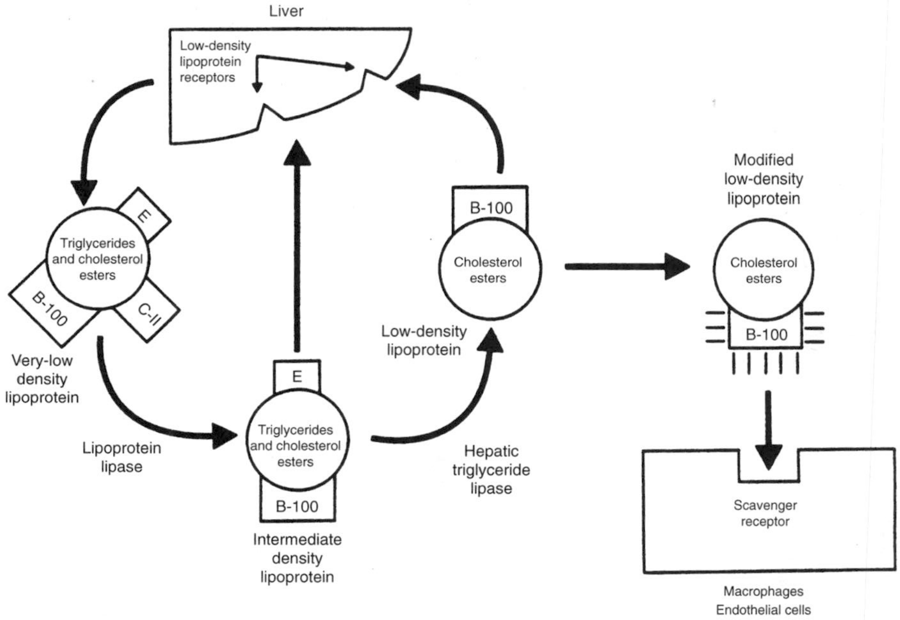

FIGURE 3.2. Endogenous fat transport. B-100 and E are apolipoproteins and bind with specific liver receptors. The liver uses large amounts of cholesterol for the manufacture of bile. Any condition or therapy that reduces the liver's supply of cholesterol provokes an increase in the number of LDL receptors, so that cholesterol-rich LDL is removed from the circulation, thus meeting the liver's needs. (Reproduced by permission from Breslow JL. Lipoprotein metabolism. Cardiol Board Rev 1989;6: 10–15.)

into the circulation. This is bound to albumin and then cleared from the circulation by the liver, which uses it as fuel.

The unused fatty acid is converted to triglyceride, which is packaged into lipoprotein particles of very low density (VLDL). Note this parallel between the exogenous and endogenous pathways: The bulk of lipid at the origin of the cascade is triglyceride, and the lipoprotein particle carrying it is large and has low density.

The triglyceride in VLDL, like that in chylomicrons, is hydrolyzed by lipoprotein lipase to free fatty acids that melt away from the particle. As with the exogenous pathway, apoC-II acts as a cofactor for lipoprotein lipase. The resulting particle is smaller, has less triglyceride, and proportionately more cholesterol and is called intermediate-density lipoprotein (IDL). This can be cleared by the liver, which has receptors for the apoE surface protein of IDL. IDL particles that are not thus removed undergo further hydrolysis to become LDL.

LDL has almost no triglyceride, and its lipid core is composed predominantly of cholesterol esters The surface protein molecule is apoB-100. LDL is the lipoprotein most commonly linked to premature atherosclerosis.

Regulation of LDL levels depends on the balance between production (via the lipolytic cascade described above) and clearance. Clearance of LDL is governed by the number of hepatocyte LDL receptors. apoB-100 on the surface of the LDL particle binds to the LDL receptor, and the LDL particle is thus absorbed by the hepatocyte.

An excess of free cholesterol within the liver cell blocks the production of LDL receptors, so that less LDL cholesterol is cleared from the circulation. A deficiency of intracellular cholesterol provokes a compensatory increase in the number of LDL receptors. More receptors ("upregulation") are able to react with LDL particles, increasing clearance of LDL from the circulation. The final common pathway for treatments to reduce LDL is the upregulation of LDL receptors (Fig. 3.3). For example, decreasing cholesterol availability by dietary restriction or by blocking an enzyme in the cholesterol synthetic pathway (HMG-CoA reductase) both cause a "deficiency" of intracellular cholesterol. The hepatocyte compensates by upregulating LDL receptors, and there is increased clearance of LDL particles from the circulation. This is a desirable result, because it is *circulating* LDL cholesterol that is atherogenic.

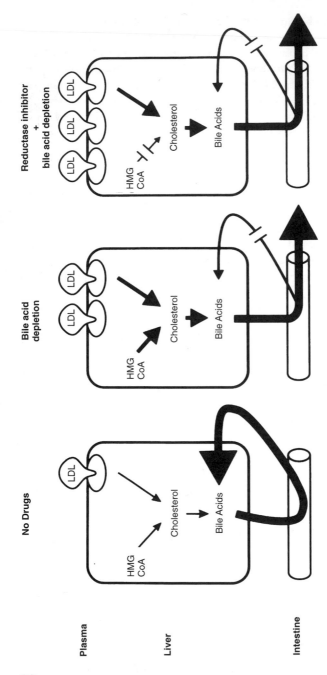

92

HDL and Reverse Cholesterol Transport

Cholesterol that is not metabolized by peripheral tissue is excreted by the liver in bile. The reverse cholesterol transport system is responsible for moving the excess cholesterol from the periphery to the liver so that it can be converted to bile (Fig. 3.4). HDL is the transport vehicle.

Production of HDL begins with secretion of apoA-I by both the liver and intestine. apoA-I complexes with phospholipid, forming a disklike structure called *nascent HDL*. This particle attracts free cholesterol from the cell membranes of peripheral tissue or from other lipoprotein particles. Free cholesterol contained in early atherosclerotic plaque may be absorbed by the nascent HDL particle.

At this stage an important enzyme, *lecithin cholesterol acyltransferase*, esterifies the free cholesterol. The cholesterol ester is less soluble than free cholesterol and moves to the inside of the phospholipid disk, which then assumes a spherical shape, is more stable, and is known as HDL. The HDL particle continues to accumulate cholesterol, not just from peripheral tissue but also from the surface of chylomicrons and from VLDL.

The liver does not have an HDL receptor. Instead, a circulating cholesterol transport protein passes the cholesterol in the particle to LDL or IDL, which is removed by the liver, or to VLDL, which is subsequently converted to LDL (Fig. 3.3). Thus, freed of its cholesterol load, the HDL particle moves on to scavenge more free cholesterol from peripheral tissue.

The level of HDL, expressed as mg/dL cholesterol by your clinical laboratory, is much lower than the level of LDL cholesterol. This gives the impression that the cholesterol removal system is comparatively small. But the HDL particle is composed of

---

FIGURE 3.3. How cholesterol-lowering therapy works. The final common pathway is reduced cholesterol availability to the liver, which increases the number of hepatocyte LDL receptors so that cholesterol can be extracted from the circulation. This happens with a low-cholesterol diet. Bile acid binding resins block the enterohepatic circulation of bile, a cholesterol-rich substance (middle panel). Reductase inhibitors block cholesterol synthesis in the hepatocyte. The combination of reductase inhibitors with either resins or diet therapy is synergistic. (Reproduced by permission from Brown MS, Goldstein JL. A receptor-mediated pathway for cholesterol homeostasis. Science 1986;232:34–47.)

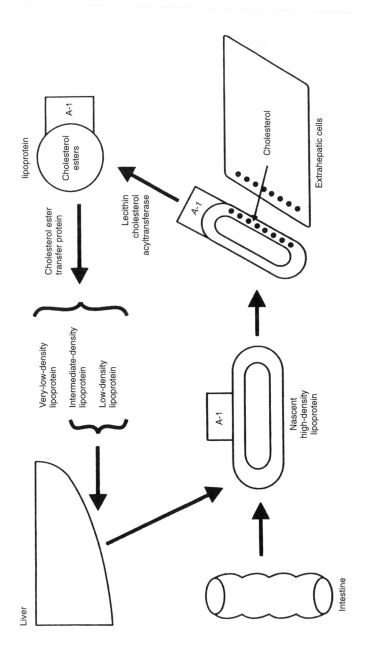

94

just 22% cholesterol, and remember that the laboratory measures just the cholesterol component of HDL. Furthermore, the HDL particle is small, weighing about one tenth of the LDL particle. In reality, the number of HDL particles (and the molar concentration) exceeds that of LDL. The total surface area of HDL particles exceeds that of all other lipoproteins. The cholesterol removal system is thus quite large.

Lipoprotein(a)

Lp(a) accounts for a small percentage of plasma cholesterol and has a density similar to HDL. Most studies have identified high levels as a risk factor for atherosclerosis that is independent of other lipoproteins. In combination with elevated LDL, high Lp(a) is especially malignant.

The apoprotein of Lp(a) is unique, having a structural subunit that is homologous to the kringle structure of plasminogen. It is tempting to speculate that this feature increases the particle's affinity for injured vascular endothelium, making it an especially efficient delivery vehicle for cholesterol into plaque.

Treatment of Hyperlipidemia

The NCEP guidelines (Table 3.5) summarize the indications for treatment and represent the standard of care. Weight reduction and reduced fat intake are the first steps in treatment.

When there is known vascular disease or diabetes, the goal of therapy is an LDL cholesterol below 100 mg/dL. This usually requires treatment with a reductase inhibitor. Achieving this goal halts the progression of disease for most patients, and the angiographic trials suggest that it may lead to regression of disease for some (Table 3.5). In addition to the long-term effects of low LDL on atherogenesis, some trials have reported fewer acute vascular events *in the short term,* before there can be an effect on plaque accumulation. The best explanation for this is that oxidized LDL is toxic enough to destabilize plaque, possibly roughening the surface

FIGURE 3.4. Reverse cholesterol transport (see text). The nascent HDL particle draws cholesterol from extrahepatic cells (including the vascular endothelium) and transfers it to VLDL and then LDL particles, which are taken up by the liver. (Reproduced by permission from Breslow JL. Lipoprotein metabolism. Cardiol Board Rev 1989;6:10–15.)

TABLE 3.7. Drug Treatment of Hyperlipidemia

Lipid Abnormality	Treatment
High LDL cholesterol	1) Reductase inhibitor—blocks cholesterol synthesis, and the liver increases the number of LDL receptors to pull cholesterol from the circulation.
	2) Niacin—highly effective (a "perfect drug" that lowers LDL and triglycerides and raises HDL) but with problematic side effects. Effective dose is ≥3 g/day.
	3) Resin—minimal reduction of cholesterol, though effective in large clinical trials (Table 3.4). Effective when combined with reductase inhibitors.
High triglycerides	When isolated, no specific treatment needed. If very high (>1000) treat with fibric acid derivatives to prevent pancreatitis (e.g. gemfibrozil). Other possibilities: niacin and fish oil. Note: many cases are secondary to high alcohol intake, diabetes, or obesity—diet modification may work.
Low HDL	No specific therapy is indicated for isolated low HDL. Niacin and fibric acid derivatives may raise it. First try exercise and a glass of wine a day (though I would not ask a nondrinker to take it up).
Combined hyperlipidemia (high LDL and VLDL and low HDL)	The major goal is reduction of LDL (using reductase inhibitors as above). Aggressive diet therapy for high VLDL (which is responsible for the high triglycerides—recall that VLDL contains a lot of it), and add exercise to raise HDL.
High Lp(a)	The first step is reduction of LDL (many recommend pushing it to ≤85 mg/dL). An occasional patient will have the Lp(a) fall with niacin.

so that platelets are activated. Reducing total LDL reduces a plaque's exposure to oxidized LDL.

The atherogenic effect of LDL cholesterol is so strong that its reduction minimizes the risk of other lipid disorders. Thus, for a patient with low HDL or another with high Lp(a), the first goal of treatment is lowering the LDL. In fact, if you remember nothing else about the treatment of dyslipidemia, keep in mind that you will usually be right if you recommend lowering LDL for any high-risk patient.

That goes for the familial dyslipidemic syndromes (Table 3.6). They are of scientific interest, but in practice you may treat dyslipidemia without a genetic diagnosis. Treatment is determined by the lipid fraction that is elevated, and the simple principles of drug therapy are listed in Table 3.7.

SUGGESTED READING

American Heart Association. Heart and Stroke Facts: 1998 Statistical Supplement. Dallas, American Heart Association, 1998.

Blankenhorn DM, Nessim SA, Johnson RL, et al. Beneficial effects of combined colestipol-niacin therapy on coronary atherosclerosis and coronary venous bypass grafts. JAMA 1897;257: 3233–3240.

Boushey CJ, Beresford SA, Omenn GS, Motulsky AG. A quantitative assessment of plasma homocysteine as a risk factor for vascular disease: probable benefits of increasing folic acid intake. JAMA 1995;274:1049–1057.

Braunwald E. Cardiovascular medicine at the turn of the millennium: triumphs, concerns and opportunities. N Engl J Med 1997;337:1360–1369. (The big picture.)

Brown G, Albers JJ, Fisher LD, et al. Regression of coronary artery disease as a result of intensive lipid-lowering therapy in men with high levels of apolipoprotein B. N Engl J Med 1990;323: 1289–1298. (As apoB is a part of the LDL particle, these patients had high LDL cholesterol levels.)

Canner PL, Berge KG, Wenger NK, et al. Fifteen-year mortality in coronary drug project patients: long term benefit with niacin. J Am Coll Cardiol 1986;8:1245–1255.

Carney RM. Psychological risk factors for cardiac events: could there be just one [Editorial]? Circulation 1998;97:128–129.

Collins R, Peto R MacMahon S, et al. Blood pressure, stroke and coronary heart disease. Part 2. Short-term reductions in blood pressure: overview of randomised drug trials in their epidimiological context. Lancet 1990;335:827–834.

Dawber TR, Meadors GF, Moore FE Jr. Epidemiologic approaches to heart disease: the Framingham Study. Am J Public Health 1951;41:279–286. (A classic reference—there are plenty of review articles and texts that describe the Framingham result, but this is an early description.)

Frick MH, Elo O, Haapa K, et al. Helsinki heart study: primary-prevention trial with gemfibrozil in middle-aged men with dyslipidemia. N Engl J Med 1987;317:1237–1245.

Gupta S, Camm AJ. Chronic infection in the etiology of atherosclerosis—the case for chlamydia pneumoniae. Clin Cardiol 1997; 20:829–836.

Hurt RD, Sachs DPL, Glover ED, et al. A comparison of sustained-release bupropion and placebo for smoking cessation. N Engl J Med 1997;337:1195–1202.

Knopp RH. Drug treatment of lipid disorders. N Engl J Med 1999;341:498–511. (In addition to a clear description of mechanisms, he nicely summarizes side effects and drug interactions. An excellent basic reference with 138 cited papers.)

Levy D, Garrison RJ, Savage DD, et al. Prognostic implications of echocardiographically determined left ventricular mass in the Framingham Heart Study. N Engl J Med 1990;322:1561–1566.

Lipid Research Clinics Program. The LRC Primary Prevention Trial results. I. Reduction in the incidence of coronary heart disease. JAMA 1984;251:351–364.

Lipid Research Clinics Program. The LRC Primary Preventions Trial results. II. The relationship of reduction in incidence of coronary heart disease to cholesterol lowering. JAMA 1984;251:365–374.

Montague T, Tsuyuki R, Burton J, et al. Prevention and regression of coronary atherosclerosis. Is it safe and efficacious therapy? Chest 1994;105:718–726.

Multiple Risk Factor Intervention Trial Research Group. Mortality rates after 10.5 years for participants in MRFIT. JAMA 1990;263:1795–1801.

Pederson TR, and the 4S Study Investigators. Randomised trial of cholesterol lowering in 4444 patients with coronary heart disease: the 4S study. Lancet 1994;344:1383–1389.

Reaven GM. Role of insulin resistance in human disease (Syndrome X): an expanded definition. Annu Rev Med 1993;44:122–131.

SHEP Cooperative Research Group. Prevention of stroke by antihypertensive drug treatment in older persons with isolated systolic hypertension: final results of the Systolic Hypertension in the Elderly Program (SHEP). JAMA 1991;265:3255–3264.

Shepherd J, Cobbe SM, Ford I, et al. Prevention of coronary heart disease with pravastatin in men with hypercholesterolemia. The West of Scotland Prevention Study. N Engl J Med 1995;333:1301–1307.

Smoking Cessation Clinical Practice Guideline Panel. The Agency for Health Care Policy and Research Smoking Cessation Clinical Practice Guideline. JAMA 1996;275:1270–1280.

Tepel M, van der Giet, Schwarzfeld C, et al. Prevention of radiographic-contrast-agent-induced reductions in renal function by acetylcysteine. N Engl J Med 2000;343:180–184. (The antioxidant worked, indicating that reactive oxygen species also have a role in the pathogenesis of contrast nephropathy [their dose was acetylcysteine 600 mg twice daily, the day before and the day of the angiogram]. Free radicals are produced when adenosine is metabolized to xanthine. Blocking the adenosine receptor with theophylline blocks renal vasospasm, but does not lower the adenosine level.)

Usher BW, O'Brien TX. Recent advances in dobutamine stress echocardiography. Clin Cardiol 2000;23:560-570. (Summarizes data comparing different imaging techniques.)

Weitz JI, Bates SM. Beyond heparin and aspirin: new treatments for unstable angina and non-Q wave myocardial infarction. Arch Intern Med 2000;160:749–758. (In addition to reviewing the latest trials, there is a concise review of how platelets contribute to plaque instability.)

CHAPTER 4

Angina Pectoris

STABLE ANGINA PECTORIS _____

More than 3 million people visit emergency rooms in the United States each year because of chest pain. Because it is so common, most who practice general medicine become adept with the differential diagnosis of chest pain (Table 4.1). An immediate goal is the recognition of cardiac pain, because heart disease can be fatal and most other causes of chest pain are not.

"Angina" comes from the Latin term with the same spelling. When used alone, it originally meant an inflammatory affliction of the throat such as quinsy. "Angina pectoris" is more specific for the chest discomfort of myocardial ischemia, but we follow the common practice of using "angina" alone. Etymologically related is "anguish," defined as an agonizing pain of body or mind. The related French word, *angoisse,* means choking, and the Latin word, *angustia,* means tightness or narrowness. All of these describe the symptom. Angina is not a superficial, fleeting, or stabbing pain. Rather, it is a deep, choking, tight discomfort with elements of agony and anguish—even though patients commonly say they "have no pain."

The onset of angina is gradual, and it mounts in intensity (by contrast, the pain of proximal aortic dissection is at peak severity at its onset). The location is usually midchest with or without radiation to dermatomes C2 to T12. When the patient points with one finger to the left side of the chest indicating pain "over my heart," it is less likely to be cardiac. Angina may have a vague quality, and there is relief over a period of minutes with rest or nitroglycerin therapy.

However, the history may be misleading. Symptoms that indicate a cardiac origin of pain may occur in those without ischemia. Similarly, atypical chest pain may be angina. Although

TABLE 4.1. Chest Pain Syndromes

Syndrome	Associated Conditions	Physical Examination	Laboratory Evaluation
Chronic stable angina	Risk factors for coronary disease (Chapter 3)	Usually normal, S_4 gallop or soft systolic murmur during pain	ECG often normal; new ECG changes during pain; abnormal stress study
Unstable angina	As above	As above	As above
Aortic dissection	Hypertension, other risk factors for coronary disease; connective tissue disease	Unequal or missing pulses, murmur of aortic regurgitation with proximal dissection	Chest x-ray (wide mediastinum), echocardiogram, CT or MRI studies, angiography
Esophageal reflux and spasm	Advanced age, often smoking and obesity	Normal	Endoscopy, pH monitoring, motility studies, barium studies
Esophageal rupture	Follows severe vomiting	Subcutaneous emphysema	Chest x-ray (air in the mediastinum)
Pancreatitis	Alcoholism, gallbladder disease	Epigastric tenderness	Elevated amylase, lipase, and white count
Peptic ulcer disease	Possibly smoking	Epigastric discomfort	Endoscopy, barium studies
Chest wall pain	Osteoarthritis, chronic back and neck pain	Pain with deep palpation, stretching, or change in position	None; usually a diagnosis of exclusion
Herpes zoster	Advanced age, immunocompromised host (but may develop in healthy young patients), prior history of shingles	Pain may precede the typical rash by 48–72 hr; rash is maculopapular, then vesicular; lesions usually few in number	Tzanck smear of a lesion, fourfold rise in antibody titer (acute vs. convalescent)
Pericarditis	Often follows a flulike illness in young patients	Friction rub; occasionally fever	High sedimentation rate; white cell count usually normal; echocardiogram

textbooks confidently recite the characteristics of ischemic discomfort, and I have heard lecturers tout the specificity of the anginal history, most of us in clinical practice are used to being fooled.

Symptoms that point to noncardiac illnesses seem more reliable and, when clearcut, exclude angina pectoris. For example, pleuritic chest pain indicates an inflammatory condition, not angina. A description of reflux esophagitis—particularly pain when recumbent, an associated sour taste, occurrence after meals, and relief by sitting upright—make angina unlikely. A musculoskeletal etiology is indicated by discomfort that occurs with movement—reaching, twisting, or use of a limb—or by reproduction of the pain by pressing on the chest wall. When sure of one of these non-cardiac illnesses, I do not pursue a cardiac workup.

Natural History

The clinical definition of chronic stable angina is exercise-induced angina for more than 2 months that is relieved within minutes by rest or nitroglycerin and that has not recently changed in frequency or severity. Stable angina tends to be stable. In the absence of left main coronary stenosis, the mortality rate is about 3% per year. Interestingly, the number of anginal episodes per week is not related to prognosis, as long as the spells are exercise induced and brief (i.e., they fit the "stable angina" pattern). Other clinical features of the disease influence prognosis:

1. *More extensive coronary artery disease (CAD) indicates a worse prognosis.* Natural history studies of patients treated medically in the 1970s found annual mortality rates of 2% to 3% with single-vessel CAD, 4% to 6% with two-vessel CAD, and 7% to 10% with three-vessel disease. The annual mortality risk is lower with modern medical therapy, particularly with antiplatelet drugs, beta blockade, and aggressive lipid lowering. Tight (>70%) left main coronary stenosis is especially dangerous, with more than 50% 1-year mortality, and exclusion of left main disease is a goal of early evaluation.

2. *Exercise tolerance determined with treadmill testing correlates roughly with survival.* Patients who have to stop the exercise test before completing stage 2 in the Bruce protocol (Table 4.2) have a 6% to 10% annual mortality, whereas those reaching stage 4 have a mortality risk of about 1% per year. A patient with poor exercise tolerance because of ischemia should be considered for angiography, and good exercise tolerance would make us more comfortable with a trial of medical therapy. For screening tread-mill studies using the Bruce protocol, 7 to 9 minutes on the treadmill (depending on age) establishes a good prognosis, inde-pendent of electrocardiographic (ECG) changes.

3. *Patients with poor left ventricular (LV) function have a bad prognosis.* This is an important principle that applies to most adult

TABLE 4.2. Bruce Exercise Test Protocol
(The patient walks in each stage for 3 min.)

Stage*	Treadmill Setting Speed	Treadmill Setting Grade	METS	Exercise Equivalent
1	1.7 mph	10%	5	5 METS is the average peak cost of activities of daily living (walking upstairs, sex with a spouse). It is the exercise limit recommended on discharge after MI.
2	2.5 mph	12%	7	
3	3.4 mph	14%	9.5	An ability to exercise to the patient's level indicates a good prognosis, even in those with known CAD.
4	4.2 mph	16%	13	This is the average peak exercise capacity for moderately active young men.

*MET is the energy equivalent of sitting quietly at rest; at this baseline the average oxygen consumption is 3.5 L/kg/min. MI, myocardial infarction.

cardiac illnesses and to those with stable angina. Defining LV function is an important part of the initial evaluation. Conditions that point to LV dysfunction include a history of myocardial infarction, Q waves on the ECG, or symptoms of congestive heart failure including easy fatigue. These clinical findings or poor LV function identified by noninvasive testing weigh in favor of angiography, even when the anginal pattern is stable.

Pathophysiology

If a machine has a plugged fuel line or a bad fuel filter, it runs smoothly when idling or at low speeds (workloads). When the throttle is opened—attempting to increase the workload—the engine begins to miss. Fuel supply is not able to keep up with fuel demand. That is the hydraulics of stable angina (Fig. 4.1).

Anginal Threshold, Stable vs. Unstable Angina

It is useful to think of stable and unstable angina as different clinical syndromes, because the pathophysiology and prognosis are different (Table 4.3). Both are caused by a coronary artery stenosis. With stable angina, the stenosis is "fixed" and does not vary. The initiating event is an increase in cardiac work, which is proportional to the heart rate multiplied by the systolic blood pressure (the "rate–pressure product"). The *angina threshold,* or the rate–pressure product at which ischemia develops, is constant. A

FIGURE 4.1. When myocardial oxygen demand (MVO_2) exceeds supply, angina develops. In chronic stable angina, the unchanging stable stenosis places a ceiling on blood supply, preventing an adequate increase in flow with increased cardiac work (a lesion is usually flow restricting when it reduces the diameter of the vessel ≥ 70%). Unstable coronary syndromes are caused by dynamic variable stenoses, either from thrombus or spasm. A failure of peripheral coronary vasodilatation, reduced oxygen-carrying capacity of blood, and low coronary perfusion pressure all may aggravate undersupply. Increased oxygen demand is the result of conditions that increase heart rate, myocardial contractility, or left ventricular wall tension.

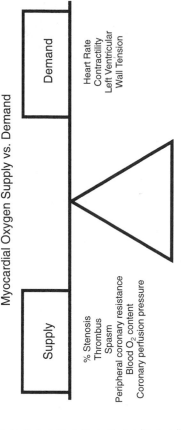

Myocardial Oxygen Supply vs. Demand

Supply

% Stenosis
Thrombus
Spasm
Peripheral coronary resistance
Blood O_2 content
Coronary perfusion pressure

Demand

Heart Rate
Contractility
Left Ventricular
Wall Tension

TABLE 4.3. Classification of Angina Pectoris

	Stable Angina	Unstable Angina
Clinical syndrome	Angina at a predictable level of exertion (the "angina threshold"). Relief with rest and nitroglycerin. No change in the anginal pattern for ≥2 months.	Any of the following: 1. New onset angina (<2 mo)* 2. Accelerating pattern 3. Angina at rest 4. Nocturnal angina 5. Long episodes of pain 6. New ST-T wave changes on the ECG
Prognosis	Annual mortality is 3–4%, and the short-term risk of MI is low.	10–20% chance of MI or death within 3–4 mo
Coronary artery lesion	Flow-restricting stenosis, but smooth plaque surface.	Stenosis, but not invariably tight. An unstable plaque surface with ulceration, exposed collagen, and possibly thrombus.

*There are varying degrees of "instability." Those with onset of angina within 2 months but who have not had angina in the previous 2 weeks and who do not have new ECG changes are "less unstable" and may be considered for exercise testing. On the other hand, those having angina within recent days or who have new ECG changes may have a preinfarction syndrome and should have angiography.
MI, myocardial infarction.

patient who gets angina after 6 minutes on the treadmill today will get it after 6 minutes on the treadmill next week, and at the same rate–pressure product. The coronary artery stenosis may be tight, but it tends to be stable, with a smooth plaque surface.

The initiating event in *unstable angina* is a drop in blood supply rather than an increase in cardiac work. The coronary artery lesion varies—and with it, blood supply—either because of thrombus on the surface of ulcerated plaque or spasm (Fig. 4.1). Continuous ECG monitoring would document ST segment changes with pain at rest, and without a preceding increase in the heart rate and/or blood pressure. Exercise stress testing may not be as useful in unstable angina; if there is no spasm or thrombus at the time of exercise, there may not be enough baseline stenosis to cause ischemia. Anatomically, the coronary lesion with unstable angina often is ulcerated, with a ragged and apparently thrombogenic surface. This is consistent with the dynamic nature of the lesion.

Physical Examination
In the absence of active ischemia, most patients with stable angina have a normal cardiac examination. Chronic ischemia or

prior ischemic injury may cause an increase in LV stiffness and an S_4 gallop.

If a patient is having chest pain, listen to the heart while you are waiting for the nurse to bring nitroglycerin. A new S_4 gallop (increased LV stiffness) or a new soft systolic murmur (transient papillary muscle dysfunction), would be objective evidence for ischemia. After angina is relieved, listen again to show that these changes have resolved.

The remainder of the physical examination is directed to possible findings of generalized atherosclerosis: depressed peripheral pulses, carotid bruit, corneal arcus, and the skin and tendon changes of hyperlipidemia.

Laboratory Testing
Noninvasive Screening for CAD

The usual resting ECG is normal. An ECG during angina is abnormal in a high percentage of patients. That is why patients in the hospital or in the emergency room with a chest pain diagnosis should have a prompt ECG with development of pain; no change in the ECG during pain makes ischemia less likely (this is not perfect, but it is a pretty good test). *Make a note on the ECG tracing that it was obtained during pain.*

The coronary arteries are on the epicardial surface of the heart, and they send perforating branches into the myocardium. Exercise-induced ischemia first affects the myocardial region farthest from the epicardial arterial source, the subendocardium. Thus, angina usually produces the ECG pattern of subendocardial ischemia, ST segment depression (Fig. 4.2). Occasionally, there will be T wave inversion, but ST depression is the common pattern of exercise-induced ischemia.

The treadmill ECG is a straightforward test. The goal is to provoke ischemia in a controlled setting so that both the symptoms and ECG might be evaluated. Be aware that the test is not 100% sensitive. I have nightmares about the patient with a normal stress test who has a myocardial infarction the next week. The test is positive only when there is a tight stenosis, which is the usual case with stable exercise-induced angina. It is not necessarily the case with unstable angina or angina at rest, where the lesion may be dynamic. Exercise testing is less accurate with unstable coronary syndromes.

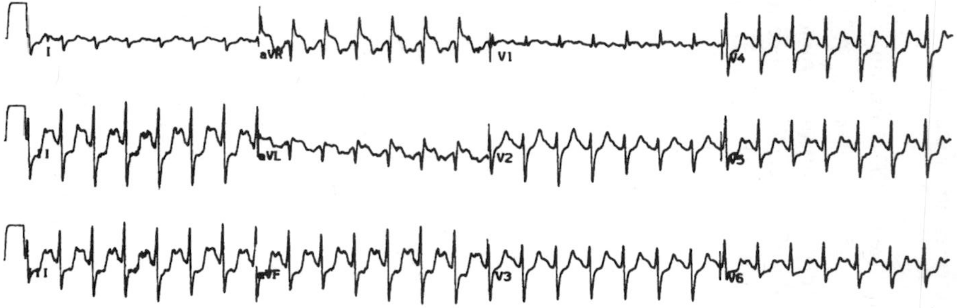

FIGURE 4.2. Positive stress ECG showing ST segment depression in inferior and lateral leads, the pattern of subendocardial ischemia (also see Fig. 5.1).

Thallium-201 enters the myocyte via the Na^+, K^+-ATPase pump and emits radiation that is detected by a gamma camera. It follows potassium and may be thought of as an intracellular cation. About 85% of injected thallium is extracted with the first pass, and myocardial accumulation is proportional to myocardial blood flow. A normal scan shows homogenous uptake by all LV segments (or "vascular distributions"). With ischemia there is a "cold spot" on the scan in the distribution of the stenosed or occluded coronary artery.

There is continuous exchange of ^{201}Tl across the membrane. With time, ischemic muscle that is viable slowly accumulates the isotope. Thus, an ischemic but viable region has a perfusion defect on the initial images but apparently normal uptake of thallium on delayed images 2–4 hours later (this filling in of an initially ischemic region is also called "redistribution" of thallium). On the other hand, scar tissue is unable to accumulate thallium, the defect does not fill in with time. Serial scans are thus able to distinguish between ischemic live muscle (a "reversible" defect) and scar (a persistent defect).

Sestamibi is another perfusion imaging agent. It is a technetium-99m compound that binds to mitochondria and is not transported by the Na^+, K^+-ATPase pump. There is rapid initial uptake, but no late redistribution into ischemic but viable muscle. Instead, the patient has an injection and scan during exercise and has a separate injection and scan done at rest. A viable region supplied by a critically stenosed artery would have a defect on the exercise images but normal uptake on the rest images.

Viability study: An occasional patient with a persistent ^{201}Tl defect on the 2–4 hour delayed image actually has viable muscle in the region. Normalization of thallium uptake on even later images, 24 hours later, indicates viable muscle. The delayed scan, viability study is done to distinguish "stunned or hibernating" myocardium from scar.

Perfusion imaging using either thallium or sestamibi increases both the sensitivity and specificity of exercise testing for flow-restricting coronary lesions (see Box 4.1). It is rare to have a false-negative scan, and the "event rate" (myocardial infarction or cardiac death) during the year after a negative scan is in the 1% range. Perfusion imaging adds more than accuracy, because the scan allows identification of the specific myocardial region responsible for ischemia.

A stress echocardiogram also raises the sensitivity and specificity of exercise studies and is able to identify the ischemic region. There is prompt cessation of contractility when muscle becomes ischemic; a new "regional wall motion abnormality" develops. The radionuclide angiogram, or "MUGA scan," can be used to assess wall motion before and during exercise as well. With both LV function and perfusion imaging techniques, the larger the ischemic region, the worse the prognosis. Anterior wall ischemia tends to be more dangerous than inferior or lateral wall defects, as the left anterior descending artery (the "LAD") supplies a larger amount of myocardium.

For an exercise study to be diagnostic, the patient must reach 85% of the maximum predicted heart rate (about 220 minus the patient's age). Orthopedic problems, deconditioning, and a number of other factors may limit a person's ability to achieve a diagnostic test. Pharmacologic stress testing is an alternative. The coronary vasodilators, dipyridamole or adenosine, are used with perfusion scanning (Box 4.2). They do not provoke ischemia but instead dilate all the coronary arteries. A diseased vessel dilates less than normal ones, so the postdilation images show less uptake (a cold spot) where there is stenosis. Intravenous dobutamine mimics exercise, increasing both heart rate and contractility, and may be used with both perfusion imaging and the echocardiogram.

One advantage of LV perfusion or functional imaging is that they are accurate in those with baseline ECG changes, including ventricular conduction abnormalities. The dipyridamole perfusion scan has been found more accurate than exercise perfusion scanning when there is left bundle branch block.

The newest screening test for coronary atherosclerosis is electron beam computed tomography (CT). Coronary plaque contains calcium, and this is imaged by this "fast CT" technique. Unlike other screening studies, plaque is detected even when flow is not restricted. Thus, the test may prove useful for the diagnosis of early, preclinical CAD in the person with risk factors. It is most sensitive for proximal left coronary and vein graft plaque. There are no clinical trials data to confirm the value of such knowledge. I would argue that a positive study places a person in the secondary rather than primary prevention category.

Other Laboratory Studies

As part of the routine evaluation of patients with possible angina pectoris, screen for anemia and hyperthyroidism, because both conditions may change the anginal threshold and aggravate symptoms. It is useful to know the status of LV function in a new patient with angina, because depressed LV ejection fraction (LVEF) adversely affects prognosis and thus would influence management. The absence of clinical heart failure does not guarantee normal LV function. LVEF is provided by the perfusion scan as well as the echocardiogram. A lipid profile is an important part of the baseline evaluation for anyone with vascular disease.

Coronary Angiography and Anatomy

Determining a need for coronary angiography is a common clinical issue. A patient with stable angina, good exercise tolerance demonstrated with a treadmill examination, and limited ischemia on an imaging study may not require angiography. Table 4.4 reviews indications for angiography, and the recommendations follow practice guidelines from the American Heart Association.

TABLE 4.4. Practice Guidelines for Coronary Angiography for Patients with Known or Suspected CAD

Clinical Setting	Appropriate	Equivocal	Not Indicated
No symptoms but known or suspected CAD	1. High-risk CAD based on noninvasive tests or clinical findings.* 2. Occupational hazard (heavy or dangerous work). 3. After cardiac arrest.	1. Borderline stress ECG, ischemia confirmed with noninvasive study. 2. Prior MI, normal LV function, positive but low risk stress test. 3. Before high risk surgery, after a positive stress test with imaging.	1. As a screening test without prior noninvasive testing. 2. Positive stress ECG alone, no other indication of high risk CAD.* 3. Routine follow-up after revascularization, without evidence for active ischemia.
Anginal symptoms, probable CAD	1. Circumstances listed above. 2. Unstable angina (Table 4.3). 3. Uncontrolled angina after revascularization. 4. Angina < 6 mo after angioplasty (probable restenosis) 5. Prinzmetal's angina.	1. All circumstances listed above. 2. Worsening exercise tolerance with serial stress ECG. 3. Inadequate noninvasive study.	1. Mild symptoms (angina only with marked exertion) + normal LV function, noninvasive studies indicate low risk.* 2. Patient is not a candidate for revascularization.
Atypical chest pain	1. Noninvasive study indicates high-risk CAD.* 2. Probable coronary spasm. 3. Associated LV dysfunction and suspicion of CAD.	1. Inadequate data from noninvasive study. 2. Negative noninvasive study but persistent and severe symptoms (e.g., multiple hospitalizations).	1. Previous normal coronary angiogram, no new objective evidence for ischemia.

*High risk CAD (coronary artery disease): *Clinical indicators* include a history of MI, congestive heart failure, a new heart murmur (mitral regurgitation) during angina, or symptoms of unstable angina (Table 4.3). *Noninvasive testing indicators* of high risk include a positive exercise study at low workloads, imaging studies showing anterior wall ischemia, ischemia of multiple vascular regions, or LV dysfunction.

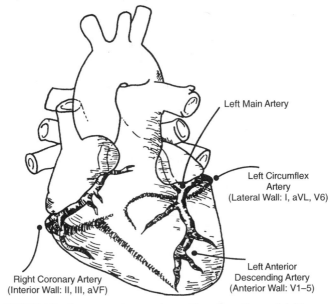

Left Main Artery

Left Circumflex
Artery
(Lateral Wall: I, aVL, V6)

Left Anterior
Descending Artery
(Anterior Wall: V1–5)

Right Coronary Artery
(Interior Wall: II, III, aVF)

FIGURE 4.3. Coronary artery anatomy. The circumflex and right coronary arteries circle the heart in the atrioventricular groove; branches of the circumflex leave the groove to supply the lateral wall of the left ventricle. The major right coronary branch, the posterior descending artery, supplies the inferior wall. The anterior descending artery is located over the interventricular septum and sends branches into the septum and over the anterior wall of the left ventricle. The spatial orientation of the ECG leads allows groups of leads to be particularly sensitive to events in a given region of the heart. This patient has a right dominant circulation, with the posterior descending branch originating from the right coronary. A small number of patients (15%) have left dominance. In this case the right coronary is tiny, and the posterior descending comes off a large circumflex vessel that reaches the base of the heart.

Coronary Anatomy

There are three major coronary artery branches (Fig. 4.3): the *left anterior descending artery,* which follows the interventricular groove and sends branches to the anterior wall and interventricular septum; the *circumflex artery,* which curls around the back side of the heart in the atrioventricular (AV) groove and reaches the lateral and posterior walls; and the *right coronary artery,* which encircles the heart in the anterior portion AV groove and has a posterior descending branch in the interventricular groove that supplies the inferior wall and basal portion of the interventricular septum.

Left main coronary disease is an indication for urgent coronary artery bypass grafting (CABG), because this trunk supplies two of the three major coronary branches. When it occludes, too much myocardium is lost and the patient usually dies suddenly. In rare cases, collateral vessels from the right coronary artery are good enough that infarction is limited and the patient survives. The left anterior descending artery supplies more muscle than other coronary branches, and for this reason left anterior descending disease is considered high risk. Anterior infarction causes more LV dysfunction than inferior or lateral myocardial infarction.

A patient has either a right or left dominant coronary circulation (Fig. 4.3). The dominant vessel is defined as the one that reaches the base of the heart in the AV groove and supplies the posterior descending branch. In 85% this is the right coronary artery. The dominant vessel also supplies the artery to the AV node; thus, AV nodal block is a common complication of inferior myocardial infarction.

LV function

Cardiac catheterization usually includes an LV angiogram, allowing measurement of LVEF. In addition, akinesis of an LV region may indicate prior infarction, usually with associated Q waves on the ECG. Hypokinesis in the absence of Q waves suggests stunned or "hibernating" muscle. Viability of an akinetic or hypokinetic segment may be further assessed using thallium perfusion imaging (stunned muscle accumulates thallium slowly, so late images show normalization of the early perfusion defect; scar tissue does not—the so-called *myocardial viability study*, Box 4.1).

Contrast Nephropathy and Other Risks

Contrast agents (or x-ray "dyes") contain iodine salts, are hyperosmolar, and have nephrotoxic effects in proportion to osmolarity. Contrast nephropathy is the leading cause of renal failure in hospitalized patients. It is worth knowing about this as a generalist, because you often send patients for angiography.

There is a tubuloglomerular reflex response to hyperosmolar stress that is largely responsible for nephropathy. It is mediated by intrarenal adenosine secretion that causes afferent arteriolar vasoconstriction and efferent vasodilatation. The net effect is glomerular ischemia. Adenosine *receptor* blockade with low-dose theophylline blunts this vasoconstrictor effect. But it does not block the release of adenosine, and intrarenal adenosine levels remain high. Recall that adenosine breaks down to xanthine and hypoxanthine. A byproduct of this reaction is the oxygen free radical, which also is a byproduct of ischemia. The free radical also provokes vasospasm and has direct nephrotoxic effects.

The best available therapy to block contrast nephropathy may include theophylline to block the adenosine receptor, plus an antioxidant to scavenge free radicals. I currently am recommending this approach: overnight hydration before angiography, Theo-Dur 200 mg the night before angiography and twice daily (bid) the day of the procedure, plus the antioxidant, acetylcysteine (Mucomyst) 600 mg bid the day of and the day following angiography. At these doses, there is little risk with prophylactic therapy. Although the combination has not been tested, clinical trials data support the use of each drug.

Other Complications of Angiography

Angiography is a relatively safe procedure, with a mortality risk of about 1 in 700, depending on the patient's condition. Other major risks are MI, stroke, and limb-threatening ischemia, all rare. It is common to see large hematoma at the catheter insertion site, especially because patients are often on antiplatelet drugs and heparin. These resolve over a period of weeks with no long-term consequence. Rarely there is *pseudoaneurysm*, a failure of the arterial puncture site to seal, with persistent communication between the arterial lumen and the hematoma. In such cases the hematoma pulsates, and there is a risk of continued bleeding, possibly into the retroperitoneal space. If there is uncertainty, the diagnosis of psuedoaneurysm can be made with an ultrasound study. Direct surgical repair of the artery is usually needed.

Management
Medical Therapy

Drug therapy of chronic stable angina is reviewed in Table 4.5. All patients with CAD should be on *aspirin,* because it has been shown to prevent myocardial infarction and improve survival. This is true also for those with coronary risk factors who do not have established CAD. The lifespan of a platelet is 9 days; stopping it 5

TABLE 4.5. Drug Therapy for Angina Pectoris

Drug	Effect on Survival	Clinical Issues Influencing Drug Choice
Aspirin	Improved (required for all with CAD).	1. May aggravate or provoke dyspepsia/ulcer 2. May aggravate asthma (especially in those with nasal polyps) 3. Clopidogrel is a substitute when aspirin is not tolerated
β-Adrenergic blockers	Improved for patients with prior myocardial infarction and for those with unstable angina. No proven benefit for others.	Negative effects 1. May provoke bronchospasm 2. May aggravate bradyarrhythmia or heart block 3. Can mask the symptoms of hypoglycemia 4. Mild worsening of dyslipidemia 5. Depression of LV contractility, aggravating heart failure 6. Can provoke coronary artery spasm and aggravate peripheral vascular disease Positive Effects 1. Good for treating hypertension 2. May prevent sudden death in those with ventricular arrhythmias 3. Improved survival for those with prior infarction 4. Also used to treat supraventricular tachyarrhythmias, tremor, migraine headache 5. Improved survival with heart failure
Nitroglycerin	None (used for control of symptoms).	1. Reduce preload may help those with heart failure and pulmonary congestion 2. Headache may preclude use 3. No negative effects on those with heart failure, bronchospasm, dyslipidemia, or diabetes

table continues

days before elective surgery ensures that most platelets will be functional at the time of the operation.

The CAPRI trial compared aspirin 325 mg/day with clopidogrel 75 mg/day for stable patients with known vascular disease and found that the risk of myocardial infarction, ischemic stroke, or vascular death was 8.7% lower with clopidogrel during 1.9 years of follow-up (5.3% vs. 5.8%). Although statistically significant in this study of 19,000 patients, I do not feel that the difference is great enough to justify switching all my patients to the more expensive drug. On the other hand, the study confirmed the safety of long-term clopidogrel therapy, and it is good to have

TABLE 4.5. *(continued)*

Drug	Effect on Survival	Clinical Issues Influencing Drug Choice
Calcium channel blockers	None.*	1. Diltiazem and verapamil slow heart rate and AV node conduction, precluding their use for some patients but favoring them for patients with supraventricular tachyarrhythmia 2. Nifedipine and amlodipine are pure vasodilators and may provoke reflex tachycardia 3. All may be used to treat hypertension (and work well for elderly patients and black patients) 4. The pure vasodilators may reduce afterload, improving heart failure, but diltiazem and (especially) verapamil depress LV contractility. 5. No adverse effects in those with bronchospasm, dyslipidemia, or diabetes 6. Effective for vasospasm, including coronary artery spasm and Raynaud's phenomenon
Lipid-lowering therapy	Lowering LDL cholesterol to <100 mg/dL slows the progression of CAD and reduces the rate of MI and cardiac death.	Most patients with high LDL require reductase inhibitor therapy (see Chapter 3).

*One clinical trial found that diltiazem reduced the chance of reinfarction for those with non-Q wave MI. There is speculation that calcium blockers that lower heart rate (diltiazem and verapamil) may be cardioprotective, but this has not been shown in patients with stable angina. MI, myocardial infarction.

it as an alternative to aspirin. (Note that CAPRI did not study the combination of aspirin and clopidogrel, which many are beginning to use for unstable coronary syndromes.)

Other than antiplatelet and lipid-lowering therapy, none of the other drugs used to treat chronic stable angina has been shown to improve survival, so the choice of initial therapy is a fielder's choice. *β-adrenergic blockers* do improve survival after myocardial infarction, and it is tempting to assume a cardioprotective effect with other coronary syndromes. For this reason many choose beta blockade as the first choice for angina, though a special benefit is unproved. Note that beta blockade does not increase coronary blood flow or change the rate–pressure product at which angina develops (the anginal threshold); rather, it lowers oxygen demand by limiting the heart rate and contractility response to exercise.

The efficacy of available beta-blockers is comparable. Relative contraindications include bronchospasm, severe LV depression, abnormalities of AV node conduction, and bradycardia. Unique properties that may influence drug choice are reviewed in Table 4.6 and may allow their use for some with relative contraindications. Mild bronchospasm, diabetes, peripheral vascular disease, and dyslipidemia would direct us to use a selective β_1 receptor agent (at low doses because selectivity is lost at higher doses). Theoretically, a patient with neurologic side effects would better tolerate a water-soluble drug that does not cross the blood–brain barrier, but I have never been impressed with this clinically. Severe hypertension may respond better to an agent with combined alpha and beta blocking activity. Resting bradycardia is not aggravated by drugs with sympathomimetic activity; during exercise when sympathetic activity increases, these drugs work like other beta-blockers, limiting the increase in heart rate.

Remember that β-adrenergic stimulation causes coronary and peripheral artery dilation, and blockade may leave alpha vasoconstriction unopposed. Thus, beta blockade may aggravate peripheral vascular disease. Beta-blocker therapy may also provoke coronary spasm. Think of this if a patient with angina gets worse with beta blockade.

Nitrates, when given at high dose intravenously, may dilate coronary arteries, but oral and cutaneous doses do not improve coronary blood flow. Instead they reduce the work of the heart by dilating peripheral veins, thus reducing blood return to the heart (or preload, see Chapter 1). An extended-release isosorbide mononitrate preparation (Imdur) provides nitrate effect for almost 12 hours. This is given in the morning and is not repeated later in the day because a 10- to 12-hour nitrate-free interval is needed to avoid *nitrate tolerance.* For the same reason, nitroglycerine patches, capable of delivering a constant dose for 24 hours, should be removed overnight.

Calcium channel blockers, unlike nitrates and beta-blockers, may improve coronary blood supply. They probably do not dilate the coronary artery at the site of stenosis but instead dilate the downstream vessel, reducing overall resistance in the system and

TABLE 4.6. β-Adrenergic Blockers with Special Properties

Property	Potential Benefit	Drugs
Cardioselective (β₁) blockade	Less bronchospasm* Less peripheral vasoconstriction.	Atenolol (Tenormin) Metoprolol (Lopressor)
Water soluble	Longer half life; do not cross the blood–brain barrier, theoretically causing fewer neurologic effects (this has not been studied).	Atenolol Nadolol (Corgard)
Intrinsic sympathomimetic activity	Less depression of heart rate at rest; at levels of higher sympathetic activity (exercise) they behave like other beta blockers.	Pindolol (Visken), Acebutalol (Sectral, a relatively weak beta-blocker)
Alpha and beta blockade	A greater antihypertensive effect.	Labetalol (Normodyne, a relatively weak beta-blocker)
Class III antiarrhythmic	Suppression of atrial and ventricular tachyarrhythmias.	Sotalol (Betapace)
Vasodilatation	The combination of beta blockade and arterial dilation is useful in heart failure.	Carvedolol

*β₂ Agonists are bronchodilators. Nonselective beta-blockers (e.g., propranolol, nadolol, and carvedolol) block both the β₁ and β₂ receptors.

improving flow. A fall in peripheral vascular resistance (LV afterload) and mild depression of contractility (with some agents) may contribute to the antianginal effect by lowering cardiac work.

There are variable effects of the calcium blockers on heart rate and contractility. The dihydropyridines are pure vasodilators and lead to reflex tachycardia (nifedipine, amlodipine, and felodipine). We no longer use the short-acting form of nifedipine, and you should not use sublingual dosing to abruptly lower blood pressure for fear of precipitating heart attack. Verapamil is a weaker vasodilator and more potently depresses contractility, heart rate, AV node conduction, and LV contraction (when there is hyperdynamic contractility, this may be attractive). Diltiazem has intermediate effects; there is some lowering of heart rate and slowing of AV node conduction, only mild depression of LV function, and moderate vasodilatation.

To summarize the medical treatment of *stable* angina, aspirin should be given to all patients with CAD, because it may prevent myocardial infarction. All patients should have aggressive lipid-lowering therapy (see Chapter 3). Despite beneficial hemodynamic effects, none of the antianginal drugs has been shown to prolong survival, and they are prescribed to control symptoms. The choice of treatment is based on other clinical features. For example, a patient with hypertension may have both angina and blood pressure controlled with beta-blockers. A person with brady-cardia or another with heart failure may have no exacerbation of these conditions with nitrates. Elderly patients seem to tolerate calcium channel blocker therapy well and often have difficulty with beta-blockers. In addition, calcium channel blockers seem effective in treating systolic hypertension in old people. Hyper-dynamic LV contraction, a possibility for those with diastolic dys-function, responds well to both beta-blockers and verapamil.

Revascularization Therapy

Clinical trials have found that revascularization improves survival when there is left main coronary disease, three-vessel CAD, and multivessel CAD plus LV dysfunction; these are broadly accepted "anatomic indications" for revascularization. As a general rule, a patient with left anterior descending coronary stenosis is consid-ered to have high-risk disease.

"Intolerable symptoms" is often the indication for angio-plasty or surgery for those with stable angina. "Intolerable" for some may be an inability to play competitive sports. On the other hand, elderly and sedentary patients may elect to live with exer-cise-related symptoms to avoid invasive treatment. Angina at a low workload, after just a couple minutes on the treadmill, is a relative indication for revascularization or at least for angiography (because it identifies poor prognosis). In practice, these indica-tions often overlap. A patient with worrisome symptoms com-monly has dangerous anatomy.

An important recent trial reported by Pitt compared medical therapy, including aggressive lipid lowering, with angioplasty for those with one- and two-vessel CAD and chronic stable angina. It found no survival advantage or reduction in the incidence of myocardial infarction with revascularization. In this study, LDL cholesterol was lowered to an average of 77 mg/dL using high-dose Lipitor. Based on this result, it appears that patients with one- or two-vessel CAD and stable angina have little to lose by trying medical therapy.

Choosing between angioplasty, with or without stenting, and CABG has become less controversial. For single-vessel disease or multivessel CAD with favorable anatomy, there is no differ-ence in survival. About 15% to 20% of patients having angioplasty have restenosis of the dilated or stented vessel and recurrence of symptoms within 6 months, and clinical trials have all found a higher incidence of repeat procedures in the angioplasty groups. That is the trade-off for avoiding surgery. Stenting of larger caliber vessel has reduced the restenosis rate. Other therapies to prevent restenosis are being tested (e.g., drug eluting or radioactive stents). Interventional techniques that "debulk" or remove plaque, either mechanical or laser atherectomy, do not lower the incidence of restenosis. Restenosis is a scarring phenomenon, and the type of initial plaque injury (mashing, burning, or cutting) apparently makes no difference.

Diabetic patients with multivessel CAD have better survival with CABG than angioplasty. Angioplasty is acceptable for single-vessel disease and a favorable lesion, but others with diabetes should have CABG. (This will likely be a board question, because it is a specific recommendation that can be derived from the clinical trials.)

UNSTABLE ANGINA PECTORIS

The clinical definition of unstable angina includes angina at rest, prolonged episodes of pain (more than 10 to 15 minutes), worsening of the angina pattern, or recent onset of symptoms (less than 2 months, Table 4.3). The term *unstable* is meaningful because the clinical syndrome is associated with a 10% to 20% risk of myocardial infarction or death within 3 to 4 months from the onset of angina. Another important clinical observation is that more than half of patients with myocardial infarction have prodromal symptoms that, in retrospect, were spells of unstable angina. In most cases they failed to recognize the discomfort as a cardiac symptom.

Some with unstable angina are more unstable than others. Findings that indicate the highest risk for myocardial infarction or early death are prolonged and ongoing chest pain, angina within the last day, new ST segment or T wave changes on the resting ECG, angina plus heart failure or hypotension, and angina with a new or worsening mitral regurgitation murmur. A common presentation is the patient with prolonged pain and new T wave inversion (changes that look like those of non-Q wave myocardial infarction) but no rise in cardiac enzymes.

Conversely, others with minimal ECG changes have a small rise in troponin or CK-MB. Both are at risk for MI.

Pathophysiology

With angina at rest, the initiating event is a reduction in oxygen supply rather than an increase in oxygen demand (Fig. 4.1). The coronary lesion is thought to be dynamic; either thrombus or spasm may lead to intermittent tightening of the stenosis and a reduction in flow. There is an anatomic correlate to instability: Instead of having smooth surfaces and a concentric hour-glass contour, the unstable coronary plaque tends to be eccentric, with a rough or irregular surface and scalloped or overhanging edges. There may be plaque ulceration or thrombus. Thrombus formation can be intermittent, with an interaction of platelets with exposed collagen on the surface of the "damaged" plaque. Platelets release vasoactive substances, provoking spasm.

Laboratory Testing

The most unstable patients should be admitted to hospital and have angiography. Myocardial infarction is excluded with cardiac enzymes and serial ECGs. An occasional patient with onset of angina within 2 months has not had pain in the last week or two and has no new ECG changes. Technically such a patient has unstable angina but is not quite as unstable as others. In such cases, screening using an exercise perfusion scan is reasonable. In one study, this subgroup with "more stable unstable angina" accounted for less than 10% of all patients with unstable angina.

It is important to screen for anemia, a potential explanation for new instability.

Treatment

As with all unstable coronary syndromes, thrombosis is key. Antiplatelet therapy with aspirin or clopidogrel is the most important treatment. Heparin is also recommended while the patient is being evaluated. More recently, the PRISM trial found the combination of aspirin plus tirofiban more effective than aspirin and heparin, underscoring the central role of platelets in the pathogenesis of unstable arterial disease. The indication for tirofiban was elevation of troponin (again, there is a blurred distinction between angina and infarction).

Beta blockade has been shown to reduce the incidence of myocardial infarction, and calcium channel blockers also may control symptoms. Intravenous nitroglycerin is especially effective in relieving pain.

Unstable angina is a common indication for revascularization when there is a tight coronary stenosis or high-risk coronary anatomy. When there is no flow restricting stenosis, or with CAD involving small coronary branches, the best choice may be medical therapy using the approach described for chronic stable angina.

LESS COMMON ANGINAL SYNDROMES _____

Prinzmetal's Variant Angina

This "variant" of angina occurs at rest and is not provoked by exercise or stress. During pain there is ST segment elevation, and angiographic study confirms coronary artery spasm as the cause. Spasm can occur at the site of atherosclerotic plaque, the case with Dr. Prinzmetal's initial cases, but also may develop in normal-appearing arteries. It may be one facet of a generalized vasospastic disorder along with Raynaud's phenomenon or migraine headache.

There is no apparent etiology for most patients. Cigarette smoking may be a risk factor. Cocaine is known to provoke spasm. It blocks the presynaptic uptake of norepinephrine and dopamine, increasing α-adrenergic tone. Similarly, β-adrenergic blockers may aggravate coronary spasm by leaving alpha stimulation unopposed. I have seen a few patients who developed Prinzmetal's angina after starting β-blocker therapy for hypertension.

Attack frequency may wax and wane, with occasional symptom-free intervals. Coronary spasm can cause myocardial infarction, which may be complicated by malignant arrhythmias (heart block or ventricular fibrillation).

Clinical Presentation

The quality of anginal discomfort is similar to that of other anginal syndromes. Pain typically occurs at rest and tends to occur at the same time each day. Nocturnal angina is common. Continuous ST segment monitoring has shown that many ischemic episodes are painless, especially when of short duration. Exercise tolerance usually is normal.

Another presentation is syncope. In these cases, patients develop ventricular tachycardia or complete heart block early during the ischemic episode, so that anginal discomfort is a less prominent symptom.

The diagnosis is confirmed when an ECG during chest pain demonstrates ST segment elevation. ST elevation is usually localized to one of the three coronary artery distributions. When ST elevation involves both anterior and inferior leads, indicating extensive ischemia, the risk of sudden death is high.

Laboratory Evaluation

An ECG during chest pain is the most useful noninvasive test and is both sensitive and specific. Patients with no ST segment changes during pain rarely benefit from angiography and provocative testing. Stress testing may be considered as a screen for underlying CAD but is of no use for the diagnosis of spasm.

Angina at rest is, by definition, unstable angina, so many of these patients have coronary angiography. It is justified when there is ST segment elevation during pain and also when there is uncertainty about the diagnosis. Angiography both confirms the diagnosis of spasm and determines the extent of atherosclerotic CAD.

Provocative testing with ergonovine maleate during angiography is the standard test for spasm. After identifying normal-appearing coronaries, the patient is given gradually increasing doses of ergonovine intravenously (from 0.05 to 0.40 mg). When angina and ST segment elevation develop, the angiogram is repeated. Spasm causes occlusion or near-occlusion of the artery. An overall reduction in coronary artery caliber without focal spasm is normal and does not indicate Prinzmetal's disease.

When angina is provoked in the catheterization laboratory, sublingual or intravenous nitroglycerin is then given for relief. An occasional patient requires intracoronary infusion of nitroglycerin. For this reason, ergonovine testing is a catheterization laboratory procedure and is never done with noninvasive techniques (echo or perfusion imaging).

The ergonovine stress test is sensitive and specific for coronary artery spasm. A normal study excludes spasm with certainty.

Those with spasm after the lowest dose of ergonovine tend to have more frequent attacks; there is a rough "dose–response" relation.

Drug Therapy

The mainstay of therapy is calcium channel blockade. These agents are so effective that I have come to think of spasm as an "illness of the calcium channel" (realizing that basic mechanisms have not been identified with certainty). All the long-acting preparations work and may need to be given at maximally tolerated doses. An occasional patient who does not respond to one of them may respond to another. A rare patient needs treatment with two different calcium blockers (from different drug classes).

There may be a rebound of symptoms when calcium blockers are stopped, such as during and after surgery. For a patient with frequent symptoms, consider intravenous diltiazem during the perioperative period.

Anginal attacks are usually relieved by nitroglycerin. In this case, it works by relieving coronary spasm. Peripheral venodilatation (reducing preload and cardiac work) is not the mechanism of action. Long-acting nitrates may be used to prevent attacks and may be used in combination with calcium blockers in resistant cases. Remember that nitrate tolerance must be avoided by providing a 10- to 12-hour nitrate-free interval. Patients who have nocturnal episodes will need to have nitrates on board overnight rather than during the day.

Spasm may be provoked by α-adrenergic discharge (e.g., the cold pressor test). A rare patient gets relief with prazosin, an appropriate drug to try if calcium blockers and nitrates fail.

Two of the standard therapies for CAD and angina may cause *worsening* of symptoms. *β-Adrenergic blockade* leaves α-adrenergic stimuli unopposed. Consider coronary spasm if your patient with hypertension develops angina after starting beta-blocker therapy. *Aspirin* inhibits synthesis of prostacyclin, a coronary vasodilator, and may thus aggrevate coronary spasm. Avoiding aspirin may help the patient with variant angina and no underlying atherosclerosis. With coronary artery plaque and spasm, benefits of aspirin may exceed risks (but monitor symptoms).

Pure vasospasm with no underlying atherosclerosis is a medical condition, not a surgical one. In fact, a failure to recognize that a stenosis is caused by spasm rather than plaque can lead to surgical disaster. Spastic arteries tend to be touchy and may develop spasm at the site of manipulation or graft insertion. Post-operative ST segment elevation, arrhythmias, and infarction may follow. On the other hand, when spasm develops at the site of a tight atherosclerotic stenosis, angioplasty with stenting or bypass surgery may be considered.

Natural History

As noted, spasm may wax and wane. The risk of myocardial infarction and death is highest for those with severe underlying atherosclerosis. Those with angiographically normal coronary arteries (pure vasospasm) have an excellent prognosis, with 5-year survival about 95% and myocardial infarction risk less than 10%.

Many patients have resolution of symptoms during the 6 months after initial presentation. It is reasonable to taper calcium blocker therapy slowly and possibly to stop it. Symptoms may recur and usually respond to the same medical regimen. I would be more concerned about stopping calcium blockers for a patient who initially presented with malignant arrhythmias. One of our patients had right coronary artery spasm and complete heart block and survived out-of-hospital cardiac arrest. Despite control of spasm with felodipine therapy, he had a pacemaker inserted prophylactically.

Syndrome X: Microvascular CAD

This syndrome has been defined as angina or angina-like chest pain with normal-appearing coronary arteries. Many of the patients included in syndrome X have noncardiac pain, but some do have microcirculatory dysfunction. About 20% have an abnormal stress test, and a smaller percentage have both ST segment changes and increased myocardial lactate production (proving ischemia) during provoked angina. In such cases, there is an apparent abnormality of coronary vasodilator reserve, because coronary blood flow does not rise with exercise or dipyridamole infusion.

A rare patient with syndrome X and objective evidence for ischemia (a positive stress test) may respond to antianginal therapy. But treating *all* patients with chest pain and normal coronary arteries with antianginal drugs will be frustrating, because most will not respond. Estrogen replacement has been found helpful in postmenopausal women with presumed syndrome X.

It is important to reassure the patient. Most with normal coronary arteries and unexplained pain have eventual resolution of symptoms. The risk of myocardial infarction or death is low. An occasional patient has persistent symptoms, with recurrent hospitalization and multiple catheterization laboratory procedures. This pattern can be avoided by using exercise imaging studies to evaluate recurrent symptoms.

Silent Ischemia

One in four patients with myocardial infarction in the Framingham study had no history of the event, and half of these had no symptoms at all. The other half could recall a prolonged episode of heartburn, indigestion, bursitis, or other discomfort that was probably the myocardial infarction. Other epidemiologic studies suggest that 2% to 4% of middle-aged men have asymptomatic but flow-restricting coronary stenoses. Patients with angina may also have silent ischemia, because ambulatory monitoring indicates that some episodes of ischemia do not cause pain. As a rule, ischemia that is longer or associated with greater ST segment shift is more likely to cause angina. This is true of variant angina with ST segment elevation and effort angina with ST depression.

Three mechanisms for silent ischemia have been proposed. The first is that a threshold quantity of ischemia must be exceeded before there is pain. The second relates to variation in pain threshold among patients. Some have a higher threshold, with a subset that produces more endorphins. The third mechanism relates to cardiac pain receptors, or nociceptive function. Patients with diabetes and neuropathy may have denervation and reduced perception of cardiac and foot pain. "Stunned nerves" may cause silent ischemia in as many as 70% of patients who have had successful reperfusion therapy for myocardial infarction. Silent ischemia is the rule after heart transplantation because of nociceptive dysfunction.

Evaluation

Silent ischemia is usually identified with stress testing. This may present a dilemma, because painless ST segment depression during exercise is one of the features that points to a false-positive study. It is usually worked out with perfusion or LV function imaging that will be abnormal during ischemia, even when silent.

Ambulatory ST segment monitoring is accurate when using systems designed for that purpose, but these are research tools. Arrhythmia detection monitors (the 24-hour Holter monitor) should not be used for the evaluation of ischemia.

Natural History and Treatment

Silent ischemia indicates an increased risk for myocardial infarction or cardiac death. When it occurs at rest, it may be considered as dangerous as other unstable angina syndromes. A special concern with silent ischemia with effort is the failure of the patient to perceive it and to stop working; the warning system is faulty.

Silent ischemia should be managed like symptomatic ischemia. Nitrates, beta-blockers, and calcium channel blockers have all been found effective. Whether the threshold for revascularization should be lower for patients with silent ischemia is uncertain at this time.

SUGGESTED READINGS _____

Chronic Stable Angina

Alexander JH, et al. for the PURSUIT Steering Committee. Association between minor elevations of creatine kinase-MB level and mortality in patients with acute coronary syndromes without ST-segment elevation. JAMA 2000;283:347–353. (A small rise in enzymes identifies the most unstable of the unstable. In other trials, such patients are selected for treatment with the newer antiplatelet drugs [see Heeschen C. Troponin concentrations for stratification of patients with acute coronary syndromes in relation to the therapeutic efficacy of tirofiban. Lancet 1999;54:1757–1762].)

Antiplatelet Trialists' Collaboration. Collaborative overview of randomized trials of antiplatelet therapy. I. Prevention of death, myocardial infarction and stroke by prolonged antiplatelet therapy in various categories of patients. Br Med J 1994;308:81–106.

Berman DS, Hachamovitch R, Kiat H, et al. Incremental prognostic value and cost implications of normal and equivocal exercise Tc-99m sestamibi myocardial perfusion SPECT. J Am Coll Cardiol 1995;26:639–647.

The Bypass Angioplasty Revascularization Investigation (BARI) Investigators. Comparison of coronary bypass surgery with angioplasty in patients with multivessel disease. N Engl J Med 1996;335:217–225.

CAPRIE Steering Committee. A randomised, blinded trial of clopidogrel versus aspirin in patients at risk of ischaemic events (CAPRIE). Lancet 1996;348:1329–1339.

CASS Principal Investigators and Their Associates. Myocardial infarction and mortality in the Coronary Artery Surgery Study (CASS) randomized trial. N Engl J Med 1984;310:750–758.

Ellis SG, Narins CR. Problem of angioplasty in diabetics. Circulation 1997;96:1707–1710.

Gibbons RJ, Chatterjee K, Daley J, et al. ACC/AHA guidelines for the management of patients with chronic stable angina. J AM Coll Cardiol 1999;33:2092. (A thorough summary of clinical trials [with 891 references]. The practice guidelines are authoritative, but be aware that new studies will influence management choices [see Pitt, below].)

Grundy SM, Balady GJ, Criqui MH, et al. When to start cholesterol-lowering therapy in patients with coronary heart disease: AHA Science Advisory. Circulation 1997;95:1683–1685.

Lewin HC, Berman DS. Achieving sustained improvement in myocardial perfusion: role of isosorbide mononitrate. Am J Cardiol 1997;79(12B): 31–35.

O'Rourke RA. Cost-effective management of chronic stable angina. Clin Cardiol 1996;19:497–501.

Pitt B, Waters D, Brown WV, et al. Aggressive lipid-lowering therapy compared with angioplasty in stable coronary artery disease. N Engl J Med 1999;341:70. (Patients with one or two-vessel CAD; those randomized to medical therapy were treated with Lipitor 80 mg/day, pushing LDL to 77 mg/dL. During 18 months of follow-up the risk of MI and death was the same in the two groups.)

Scandinavian Simvastatin Survival Study Group. Randomised trial of cholesterol lowering in 4444 patients with coronary heart disease: the Scandinavian Simvastatin Survival Study (4S). Lancet 1994;344:1383–1389.

Solomon AJ, Gersh BJ. Management of chronic stable angina: medical therapy, percutaneous transluminal coronary angioplasty, and coronary artery bypass surgery. Lessons from the randomized trials. Ann Intern Med 1998;128:216–223.

Thadani U. Management of patients with chronic stable angina at low risk for serious cardiac events. Am J Cardiol 1997;79 (12B):24–30.

Vogel RA. Coronary risk factors, endothelial function and atherosclerosis: a review. Clin Cardiol 1997;20:426–432.

Yusuf S, Zucker D, Peduzzi P, et al. Effect of coronary artery bypass graft surgery on survival: overview of 10 year results from randomized trials by the Coronary Artery Bypass Graft Surgery Trialists Collaboration. Lancet 1994;344:563–570.

Unstable Angina Pectoris

Braunwald E. Unstable angina: a classification. Circulation 1989; 80: 410-414.

Braunwald E, Mark DB, Jones RH, et al. Unstable angina: diagnosis and management. Clinical Practice Guideline Number 10 (amended). Rockville, MD: Agency for Health Care Policy and Research, 1994. Publication No. 94-0602.

Chester M, Chen L, Kaski JC. Identification of patients at high risk for adverse coronary events while awaiting routine coronary angioplasty. Br Heart J 1995;73:216–222.

Cohen M, Demers C, Gurfinkel EP, et al. A comparison of low molecular weight heparin with unfractionated heparin for unstable coronary artery disease (ESSENCE trial). N Engl J Med 1997;337: 447–452. (LMW heparin is as effective.)

Katz DA, Griffith JL, Beshansky JR, Selker, HP. The use of empiric clinical data in the evaluation of practice guidelines for unstable angina. JAMA 1996;276:1568–1574. (Only 6% of patients in this study met the Braunwald criteria for "low risk unstable angina." Most patients are in the higher risk groups and need hospital admission.)

Oler A, Whooley MA, Oler J, Grady D. Adding heparin to aspirin reduces the incidence of myocardial infarction and death in patients with unstable angina: a meta analysis. JAMA 1996;276: 811–815.

The PRISM Study Investigators. A comparison of aspirin plus tirofiban with aspirin plus heparin for unstable angina. N Engl J Med 1998;338:1498. (More aggressive antiplatelet therapy was superior to aspirin plus heparin. Arterial thrombosis is a platelet phenomenon, and the clotting cascade has a less important role.)

Shah PK. New insights into the pathogenesis and prevention of acute coronary syndromes. Am J Cardiol 1997;79(12B):17–23.

Other Reading

Achenbach S, Moshage W, Bachmann K. Noninvasive coronary angiography by contrast-enhanced electron-beam computed tomography. Clin Cardiol 1998;21:323–327. ("Ultra-fast" computed tomography has about 90% sensitivity and specificity and is best for finding calcium [plaque] in the left main and anterior descending arteries and vein grafts.)

Bennet RM. Emerging concepts in the neurobiology of chronic pain: evidence of abnormal sensory processing in fibromyalgia. Mayo Clin Proc 1999;74:385–389. (Another cause of chest pain, plus a good review of nociceptive function.)

Cannon RO. The cardiovascular syndrome X: is it real? ACC Education Highlights 1998;14:1–6. (Excellent review of what is often a bogus diagnosis.)

Katholi RE, Taylor GJ, McCann WP, et al. Nephrotoxicity from contrast media: attenuation with theophylline. Radiology 1995;195:17–22.

Parker JD, Parker JO. Nitrate therapy for stable angina pectoris. N Engl J Med 1998;338:520–531.

Tepel M, van der Giet, Schwarzfeld C, et al. Prevention of radiographic-contrast-agent-induced reductions in renal function by acetylcysteine. N Engl J Med 2000;343:180–184. (The antioxidant worked, indicating that reactive oxygen species also have a role in the pathogenesis of contrast nephropathy [their dose was acetylcysteine 600 mg twice daily, the day before and the day of the angiogram]. Free radicals are produced when adenosine is metabolized to xanthine. Blocking the adenosine receptor with theophylline blocks renal vasospasm, but does not lower the adenosine level.)

Usher BW, O'Brien TX. Recent advances in dobutamine stress echocardiography. Clin Cardiol 2000;23:560-570. (Summarizes data comparing different imaging techniques.)

Weitz JI, Bates SM. Beyond heparin and aspirin: new treatments for unstable angina and non-Q wave myocardial infarction. Arch Intern Med 2000;160:749–758. (In addition to reviewing the latest trials, there is a concise review of how platelets contribute to plaque instability.)

CHAPTER 5

Myocardial Infarction

The incidence of myocardial infarction (MI) has declined, but that of unstable angina has increased, suggesting that patients are coming to the hospital earlier with warning symptoms instead of later with infarction. Nevertheless, in 1998, 1.1 million Americans had a new or recurrent MI, and about one third of them died. About one third of the deaths occurred within 1 hour of the onset of symptoms, before reaching the hospital.

PATHOPHYSIOLOGY OF MI

An abrupt interruption of coronary artery blood flow causes contractile activity of ischemic muscle to stop within a few heartbeats. All energy is then devoted to maintaining cellular viability. During the subsequent minutes to hours, cell death occurs. Cell membrane deteriorates, and cellular contents, including contractile proteins (the "cardiac enzymes"), leach out of the infarct zone and into circulating blood.

Platelet Function and the Onset of MI

Atherosclerotic plaque is the underlying illness, but infarction is usually initiated by thrombosis. For reasons that are unclear, the lipid-rich plaque ruptures, injuring the surface of the plaque. Fissures in the surface expose collagen, and collagen is thrombogenic. Platelets adhere and are activated, release vasoactive amines, and thus promote spasm. Platelets are also rich in plasminogen activator inhibitor-1 (PAI-1), a potent inhibitor of fibrinolysis. Because of PAI-1, thrombolytic agents have less effect on platelet-rich "white clot" than they have on fibrin and red cell-rich thrombus ("red clot"). The continued activation of platelets is one reason for failure of thrombolytic therapy, and better antiplatelet adjunctive therapy is emerging as a key to improving the results of coronary thrombolysis.

It is possible for this sequence of plaque injury and thrombus formation to develop on coronary plaques that are not flow restricting. This is the usual mechanism of heart attack in the person with a recent normal stress electrocardiogram (ECG). One study of patients with MI who had angiography months to years earlier found that many " infarct arteries" (jargon for the coronary artery branch responsible for the MI) had less than 50% stenosis, suggesting a change in the plaque just before MI.

Infarct Size and Cumulative Injury

The prognosis of all patients with coronary artery disease (CAD) is most accurately predicted by left ventricular (LV) function, measured as LV ejection fraction (LVEF), and preservation of LVEF is the first goal of treatment. LVEF is the proportion (or fraction) of blood ejected by the left ventricle with each beat. Thus, when the end-diastolic LV volume is 150 mL and end-systolic volume is 50 mL, LVEF is 67%. Normal LVEF is at least 55%, with slight variation depending on the technique used to measure it.

In the absence of early reperfusion, the amount of creatine kinase (CK) released during MI is proportional to infarct size and inversely proportional to subsequent LVEF. (A caveat is that non-infarcted LV segments may compensate with hyperdynamic contraction, slightly raising the LVEF, but in general LVEF is inversely proportional to infarct size.)

Cardiac injury is cumulative. Damaged muscle is replaced by scar and never grows back. I tell patients that losing heart muscle is like losing a finger, which cannot regenerate. Thus, a person who loses 10 EF points with a first MI and later loses another 10 points must then live with an EF of no more than 35%. When a large MI or multiple infarcts push LVEF below 30%, there usually is a loss of exercise tolerance or heart failure. An LVEF < 30% is one of the Social Security Administration's criteria for cardiac disability.

Because damage is cumulative, a major treatment goal after MI is the prevention of future ischemic injury. The mortality risk with a second MI is much higher than that of the first. After any heart attack you may tell your patient, "You have lost all the muscle you can afford to lose."

TABLE 5.1. A Spectrum of Ischemic Coronary Syndromes

Syndrome	ECG Changes	Coronary Anatomy, Clinical Pattern, Enzymes
Chronic stable, exertional angina	ST segment depression during angina (usually normal between episodes).	Smooth plaque surface. No recent change in symptoms.
Unstable angina	ST segment depression with angina. If angina is caused by coronary artery spasm, there may be ST segment elevation (indicating transmural ischemia).	The ragged plaque surface is dynamic, prone to thrombosis or spasm. Pain at rest or a recent acceleration in the anginal pattern. No release of CK.
Non-Q MI ("subendocardial or nontransmural" MI)	Symmetric T wave inversion, which may or may not resolve. ST segment depression during pain.	An open but stenosed artery, with ragged plaque surface, prone to thrombosis. A modest rise in CK (confirming injury).
Q wave MI ("transmural" MI)	ST segment elevation develops immediately with occlusion. This is followed minutes to hours later by T wave inversion and Q waves.	An occluded artery, with full-thickness injury of the affected LV segment. Marked rise in CK.

Non-Q Versus Q wave MI

It is useful to think of coronary syndromes as a clinical spectrum (Table 5.1). The most stable of them is chronic exercise-induced angina. The first of the unstable syndromes is "unstable angina," usually a result of changes in the coronary artery plaque (e.g., plaque rupture, ulceration, or thrombosis, Chapter 4).

Non-Q wave MI, also called nontransmural or subendocardial MI, is the next level of instability. Early angiography has shown that the infarct artery is usually open, though tightly stenosed. The plaque surface appears ragged, scalloped, or ulcerated, and there may be thrombus (which appears as a filling defect on the angiogram). The appearance of the plaque is similar to that causing unstable angina, with ragged plaque surface.

A non-Q wave infarction causes relatively little muscle injury: the peak CK may be just two to three times normal, usually below 600 U. LVEF is either normal or minimally depressed, and there is hypokinesis (not akinesis) of the infarct zone. Injury is localized to the subendocardial region of the heart, the portion of myocardium farthest from the epicardial coronary arteries. This produces the distinctive ECG pattern of symmetric T wave inversion, possibly with ST depression during pain (Fig. 5.1).

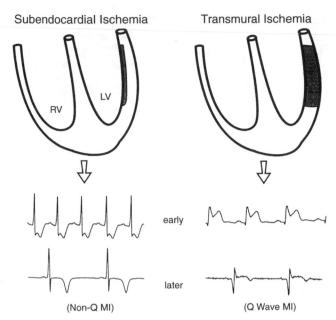

Subendocardial Ischemia   Transmural Ischemia

LV
RV

early

later

(Non-Q MI)   (Q Wave MI)

FIGURE 5.1. Patterns of myocardial ischemia. The coronary arteries rest upon the epicardial surface, and the subendocardial region is thus farthest from the source of nutrient supply. When there is tight stenosis of a coronary artery (but still some antegrade flow), a mismatch between oxygen supply and demand produces the pattern of subendocardial ischemia, ST segment depression. A good example of this is a positive stress test. Total occlusion of a coronary artery affects the full thickness of the myocardium, causing ST segment elevation, the pattern of transmural ischemia. This is usually the case with acute myocardial infarction. Note that *ischemia* does not equal *infarction*. If ischemia persists long enough to cause injury, the patterns of non-Q or Q wave infarction develop (see Table 5.1).

Your initial report to the patient with non-Q MI is optimistic: This is a small heart attack and, after all, long-term prognosis is determined by the amount of LV injury. On the other hand, non-Q MI must also be considered an "incomplete" infarction. The tightly stenosed and unstable infarct artery is at risk for thrombosis and occlusion, or "completion of the MI." We learned about this in the 1970s when multiple studies found that patients with non-Q MI had a 1-year prognosis as bad as those with larger Q wave infarction. In-hospital survival was better, but on medical therapy many of them reinfarcted soon after discharge, suffering the consequences of the larger MI. Because of this, you should consider non-Q MI a step more unstable than unstable angina. The patient should be anticoagulated and have further study before hospital discharge.

Q wave infarction begins with total occlusion of the infarct artery, transmural ischemia, and ST segment elevation on the ECG (Fig. 5.1). Later in the course of infarction, Q waves evolve. The infarction is larger with higher CK levels and a substantial fall in LVEF, particularly with anterior MI. The infarction is "complete." That is to say, there is permanent damage of all of the muscle that is susceptible to injury; recurrence of ischemia and injury in that myocardial region is not possible.

The distinction between non-Q and Q wave infarction is not 100% reliable. Some patients with transmural ischemia do not develop Q waves (usually with lateral wall MI, vide infra). Conversely, many with Q waves do not have completed transmural injury. This is common when infarction is interrupted early in its course by either thrombolytic therapy or angioplasty. In fact, rapid evolution of Q waves is characteristic of early reperfusion. *Spontaneous thrombolysis* may occur early enough to open the infarct artery and save ischemic myocardium. Regardless of whether early thrombolysis is spontaneous or drug induced, the patient is left with incomplete injury and is at risk for recurrent thrombosis and reocclusion. This is the usual mechanism of *"extension of infarction,"* the recurrence of chest pain and ST segment elevation with further injury and release of cardiac enzymes that may occur days after the initial MI.

CLINICAL PRESENTATION

Triggers of the Onset of MI

The peak incidence of MI is between 6 a.m. and noon, a pattern that coincides with an elevation of plasma catecholamines and cortisol and an increase in platelet aggregation. Patients on beta-blockers and aspirin do not exhibit this circadian variation in the timing of infarction. There are a number of well-recognized triggers of MI: heavy physical work, particularly with fatigue or exposure to environmental extremes (especially the cold); stress; anger; upsetting life events; hypoxemia; use of ergot preparations, cocaine, and other agents that may provoke coronary spasm (including β-adrenergic blockers and rarely cyclophosphamide and 5-fluorouracil); use of short-acting calcium blockers that may abruptly lower blood pressure; other illnesses (stroke, hypoglycemia, shock, sepsis); and possibly the withdrawal of beta-blocker or nitrate therapy. Sexual activity can trigger the onset of MI, but this is uncommon, occurring in less than 1% of cases.

MI develops in less than 10% of patients admitted to the hospital with unstable angina. But it is common for patients with MI to describe prodromal symptoms during the days or weeks before infarction. In retrospect, they had unstable angina.

History and Physical Examination

Abrupt occlusion of a coronary artery usually causes chest pain. The quality and location of pain is "anginal." Patients who have had angina and then develop MI usually report that the pain is recognizable as cardiac but that it is more severe. There is associated diaphoresis and a sense of impending doom. Nausea and vomiting are common, regardless of the location of MI, as is dyspnea.

Silent MI, without any symptoms, accounts for at least 10% of all cases. It is more common in those with diabetes or hypertension and in patients with no history of angina before MI. Silent MI may be followed by silent ischemia (a positive stress ECG without angina). The prognosis after silent MI is no different than with symptomatic MI.

On physical examination during MI, the patient is in obvious distress and is often restless. There usually is an S_4 gallop. A soft systolic murmur indicates papillary muscle dysfunction and mitral regurgitation, more common with inferior and lateral MI. The Killip classification is useful for defining prognosis at the time of presentation and is based on clinical evidence of LV dysfunction (Table 5.2). It is thus important to note the presence or absence of rales. Other signs of advanced LV dysfunction include an S_3 gallop and resting tachycardia (especially in the absence of severe pain).

Inexperienced clinicians often miss the importance of sinus tachycardia. When the patient is at rest and free of pain or distress, resting tachycardia is an "arrhythmia" that indicates a worse long-term prognosis than does successfully treated ventricular fibrillation (VF). It is a marker of poor LV function, and VF in the first 24 hours of MI is not.

TABLE 5.2. The Killip Classification of Heart Failure During Acute MI

Class	Mortality (%)*	Clinical Definition
I	6	No rales ("no heart failure")
II	17	Rales
III	38	Pulmonary edema
IV	81	Cardiogenic shock

*Mortality rates from Dr. Killip's 1967 study; with contemporary therapy the risk of death is lower, but the risk still parallels the severity of pulmonary congestion and LV dysfunction.

Reproduced by permission from Killip T, Kimball JT. Treatment of myocardial infarction in a coronary care unit. A two-year experience with 250 patients. Am J Cardiol 1967;20:457–464.

A transient pericardial friction rub is common during the first 3 days after transmural infarction. It is more common with large anterior MI. About 70% of patients with a rub also have pleuritic or positional chest pain. Pericarditis developing more than 10 days after MI indicates Dressler's syndrome and is thought to be autoimmune in origin.

LABORATORY EVALUATION

Cardiac Enzymes

The diagnosis of acute MI is based on a triad of chest pain, ECG changes, and a rise in cardiac enzymes. When drawn at the appropriate time, normal enzymes would make it hard to diagnose acute MI. The peak CK or the area under the CK curve is proportional to the size of infarction.

Because of the delay in CK release, there has been interest in muscle components that reach the circulation earlier after the onset of MI (Table 5.3). Smaller molecules appear earlier; myoglobin, about one fifth the weight of CK-MB, may be elevated 1 hour after the onset of chest pain. *None of the available markers is elevated at the onset of infarction. A decision about reperfusion therapy must be made based on history and the ECG.*

The other major issue with cardiac enzymes is specificity. CK-MB, cardiac specific troponins, and LDH_1 are relatively specific for myocardial damage. There is a small amount of CK-MB in skeletal muscle, and for this reason the ratio of CK-MB to total CK is reported. An occasional patient with a tiny MI will have a normal total CK but elevation of the CK-MB and the CK-MB/CK ratio. Spilling a small amount of enzyme indicates a

TABLE 5.3. Cardiac Enzymes

	Time of Appearance*		Myocardial Specific	Comment
	Earliest	Peak		
Total creatine kinase (CK)	4–8 hr	20–24 hr	No	Falls to normal in 2–3 days. False positives with muscle trauma, injections, vigorous exercise, alcohol intoxication, pulmonary embolism. Peak CK and the area under the CK curve provide estimates of infarct size.
CK-MB	4–8 hr	24 hr	Yes	The small amount of MB in skeletal muscle can cause false positives with strenuous exercise. Ratio of CK-MB/total CK > 2.5% suggests a cardiac source.
CK-MB$_2$	2–4 hr		Yes	Earlier appearance of this isoform may allow earlier diagnosis. Experimental.
Cardiac specific troponins (cTnI and cTnT)	3–12 hr	24 hr	Yes	Elevation may persist 7–14 days. Earlier appearance may help with early diagnosis. More sensitive than CK-MB.
Myoglobin	1–2 hr	1–4 hr	No	Earliest appearing, but nonspecific. Do not use to diagnose MI in absence of ECG changes.
Lactic dehydrogenase-1 (LDH$_1$)	8–24 hr	3–6 days	Yes	Total LDH is nonspecific. The heart contains LDH$_1$. Hemolysis may raise LDH$_1$. A ratio of LDH$_1$/LDH$_2$ > 1.0 is sensitive and specific for MI.

*The timing of enzyme changes in the absence of reperfusion therapy. Earliest = time from the onset of MI to the first abnormal value. Normal values vary among laboratories.

140

worse prognosis when compared with suspected MI but normal CK-MB and ratio.

Measurement of troponin is now common in community hospitals. There is a problem with false positives. Early in its use, we found that many patients with mild elevation were transferred to the referral center for angiography and were found to have no disease. On the other hand, false negatives are rare, and a negative troponin level effectively excludes MI. A pilot study found that patients with no ST segment changes on the ECG and two negative troponins, with the second measured at least 6 hours after the onset of chest pain, had an excellent 30-day prognosis. If this is confirmed by larger experience, such patients may be discharged from the emergency room rather than admitted to hospital, though with plans for early outpatient evaluation.

At this time we draw cardiac enzymes at the time of presentation and at 8-hour intervals. When there is associated skeletal muscle injury, cardiac specific troponin is especially useful.

Other Laboratory Studies

Total and high-density-lipoprotein cholesterol remain at baseline levels for 24 hours after MI. After 48 hours, both fall considerably, with high-density lipoprotein falling more than total cholesterol. For this reason, a serum lipid profile on admission or during the first day of MI is drawn. If it is not possible to get lipid studies within 2 days, wait 8 weeks to determine the baseline levels.

The white cell count begins to rise the day of infarction. It peaks at 2 to 3 days, usually around 12,000/mm^3, with a shift to the left. It may go to 20,000/mm^3 with large transmural MI. There may be low-grade fever as well. The erythrocyte sedimentation rate is normal the first couple of days, even in the face of fever and leukocytosis, and then rises and peaks on days 4 and 5. It may remain elevated for weeks.

ECG Patterns of MI

Coronary occlusion causes ST segment elevation and subsequently, T wave inversion, and Q waves (Figs. 5.1 to 5.3 and Table 5.1). The pattern of non-Q MI, caused by tight coronary artery stenosis rather than occlusion, is symmetric T wave inversion (Fig. 5.2). There may or may not be ST segment depression during pain.

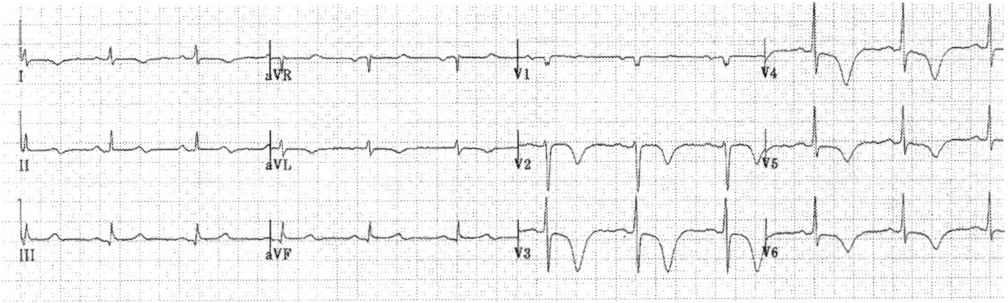

FIGURE 5.2. Anterior non-Q wave MI. There is symmetric T wave inversion in anterior precordial leads.

142

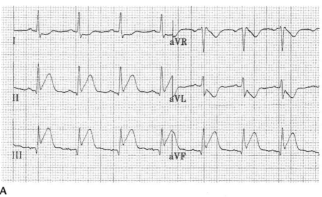

A

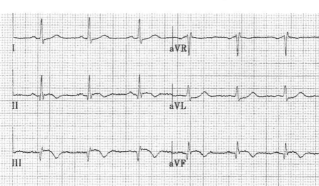

B

FIGURE 5.3. Evolution of inferior transmural MI (just the six limb leads). *Top ECG:* During the acute phase of infarction there is ST segment elevation in the inferior leads (II, III, and aVF). "Reciprocal" ST segment depression is seen in I and aVL. *Bottom ECG:* The next day there is less ST segment elevation, and the reciprocal ST depression has resolved. The T waves have inverted and deeper Q waves have evolved.

Anterior MI

Anterior transmural MI is usually the largest infarction, with the greatest rise in CK and depression of LVEF. The simple reason for this is that the left anterior descending artery, which supplies the anterior wall and the bulk of the interventricular septum, is the coronary branch supplying the most muscle (Fig. 4.3). There is variation of the size of coronary arteries from patient to patient, but as a rule, most who develop heart failure after a first infarction have had an anterior MI.

It is possible to estimate the size of the anterior MI from the initial ECG: The number of leads with ST segment elevation is proportional to peak CK and depression of LVEF. Thus, a patient with ST segment elevation in leads V_{1-3} is having a smaller MI than another with elevation in V_{2-6}.

Inferior MI

The initial ECG also provides an estimate of inferior infarct size but the criteria are different. Rather than the number of leads with ST elevation, the degree of ST elevation in the inferior leads (II, III, and aVF) is proportional to the size of MI. Thus, a patient with 3 to 5 mm of ST segment elevation in each of the three inferior leads is having a much bigger MI than another with just 1 to 2 mm of ST elevation.

"Reciprocal" ST segment depression in anterior or lateral also identifies large inferior MI. There is uncertainty about the cause of the changes. It was first described as a reciprocal electrical phenomenon (ST elevation on one side of the heart leading to depression on the opposite side). "Ischemia at a distance" has also been suggested, although patients with these changes commonly have single-vessel right coronary disease and normal blood flow to the anterior and lateral walls. Another mechanism, which I find more plausible, is that an unusually large right coronary artery also sends branches to the posterolateral wall, causing lateral ECG changes and greater CK release.

Right Ventricular Infarction Pattern

The right coronary artery supplies the right ventricular (RV) free wall as well as the inferior wall of the left ventricle and the base of the interventricular septum. Mild RV dysfunction is common with inferior MI. In some cases it is severe enough to cause RV failure and/or cardiogenic shock, referred to as the RV infarction syndrome. The ECG may have mild ST elevation in V_1, but the finding that is most sensitive and specific for RV infarction is ST elevation in V leads recorded from the right side of the chest, V_{3R}-V_{6R}. As with other inferior infarctions, there is also ST elevation in the inferior leads.

Lateral MI

The posterolateral wall of the left ventricle often is "electrocardiographically silent." Occlusion of a small circumflex artery may not cause ST segment elevation in lateral leads. Instead, there may be minimal ST depression or T wave inversion in V_{5-6}, a pattern more consistent with nontransmural ischemia, even though subsequent angiography shows circumflex occlusion and akinesis of the lateral wall. The CK usually peaks three to four times the top-normal value, higher than is usual for non-Q infarction.

Because there is no ST elevation or Q wave evolution, this technically is non-Q MI. But total occlusion of the circumflex artery and akinesis of the afflicted ventricular segment identify completed transmural infarction.

An occasional patient with lateral MI has no ECG changes at all. In fact, patients with MI and no ECG changes are usually having lateral infarction. This is the rationale for observing a patient in the hospital who has convincing chest pain but no ECG changes, at least until serial cardiac enzymes exclude MI.

Anterolateral and Inferolateral Infarction

Acute MI usually affects just one vascular distribution. It would be a remarkable coincidence for two coronary arteries, supplying two different regions, to occlude at the same time. When the distribution of infarction spills from the anterior or inferior walls into the lateral wall, it is not because a second artery has occluded. Instead, it indicates that the infarct artery—either the right or left anterior descending—is unusually large, with branches to the lateral wall.

Conduction Abnormalities and Patterns of MI

Q waves appear at the beginning of the QRS, and the initial segment of the left ventricle that is depolarized is the interventricular septum. When a conduction abnormality develops that does not disturb septal depolarization, it is possible to discern patterns of infarction. Right bundle branch block affects only the terminal half of the QRS complex and does not influence either the ST segment changes of infarction or the evolution of Q waves (Fig. 5.4).

Left bundle branch block interrupts early septal activation, which instead occurs late (toward the end of the QRS complex). In most cases it is not possible to diagnose acute MI when there is

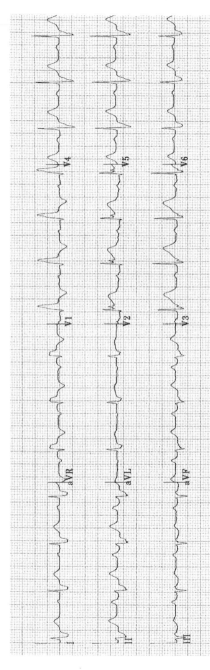

FIGURE 5.4. Acute anterior MI and right bundle branch block. The conduction abnormality does not obscure the ST elevation in leads V_{1-3}.

left bundle branch block. ST segment elevation at least 1 mm in a lead with a positive QRS complex (the vector of the ST segment and the QRS are "concordant") indicates acute ischemia. ST elevation more than 5 mm in other leads or ST depression in V_{1-3} also suggests acute MI but is a less specific finding.

Pseudoinfarction

The ST segment elevation of *pericarditis* can mimic the changes of acute transmural ischemia. Usually they are diffuse, involving both anterior and inferior leads. With persistent pain, T wave inversion may also develop. However, with pericarditis the ST segments usually return to baseline before the T waves flip; with ischemia the T waves turn over while the ST segments are still up. A rare patient with *myocarditis* has ST segment elevation, T inversion, and evolution of Q waves, a pattern indistinguishable from acute MI. There may be cardiac enzyme changes as well. Diffuse ST elevation in multiple vascular distributions suggests myocarditis, but angiography is usually needed to sort it out.

The delta wave of Wolff-Parkinson-White syndrome may appear as Q waves, usually in the inferior leads. A short PR interval points to the correct diagnosis, and it is supported by the history (no prior MI) and echocardiogram (no regional wall motion changes).

TREATMENT OF MI

The following treatment recommendations are consistent with those of the Practice Guidelines of the ACC/AHA Task Force. Most of the guidelines come from clinical trials and are thus evidence based.

The most important treatment option soon after the onset of MI is reperfusion therapy. Success depends on the rapidity of its application, and early reperfusion should be the goal of everyone taking care of the patient. Having said this, let us first review other therapies commonly used during the acute phase of MI.

Prehospital Treatment

About one third of the deaths from MI occur before the patient reaches the hospital. VF is the usual mechanism, and the risk of VF is highest during the initial 6 hours of infarction. Recognition of symptoms by the patient and early ECG monitoring is the best way to avoid death from early VF.

Treatment in the Initial 12 Hours of MI
Oxygen
There is little evidence to support its efficacy for those who do not have hypoxemia, and it is not identified as a critical therapy by the Practice Guidelines. However, patients often describe improvement in pain with oxygen treatment. Because there is little risk with nasal oxygen 2 to 4 L/min, there is no reason to omit this traditional treatment. The common practice has been to continue it for a couple days or longer. If oximetry shows normal saturation on room air, stopping it after 12 hours is sensible. Another approach would be to stop oxygen as soon as the patient is pain free and has normal arterial oxygen saturation.

Aspirin
Barring a history of drug allergy, one adult aspirin (325 mg) should be given immediately on arrival in the emergency room. In fact, this is commonly administered by the ambulance team in the field. (If your patient contacts you before calling 911, recommend an aspirin while the ambulance is on the way.) Have the patient chew the aspirin for more rapid absorption. The ISIS-2 trial reported that one chewed aspirin reduced 30-day mortality by 23%, a result similar to that achieved with intravenous streptokinase (STK), and mortality was 42% lower when aspirin was given with STK (Fig. 5.5). The remarkable effectiveness of aspirin highlights the role of platelets in the early stage of coronary thrombosis.

Control of Pain
Initial treatment of the patient with a palpable pulse and adequate blood pressure with sublingual *nitroglycerin* is fine, even before getting the ECG. If you are in fact treating angina (with an open but stenosed coronary artery) rather than MI (with an occluded artery), there may be prompt relief of pain. Hypotension after nitroglycerin usually improves with recumbency. If it persists, elevate the patient's legs.

Morphine is the preferred analgesic. Meperidine is less effective, has similar side effects, and tends to raise the heart rate more.

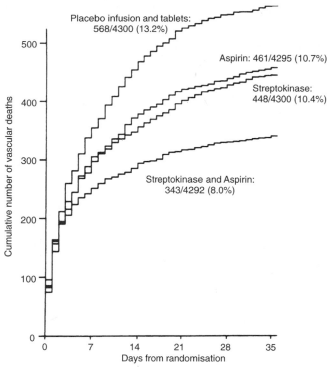

FIGURE 5.5. The ISIS-2 trial randomly assigned patients with acute MI to four groups: aspirin alone, streptokinase alone, the two together, and placebo. This classic study identified the key role of platelets in the pathogenesis of acute MI.

Like nitroglycerin, morphine is a venodilator and thus lowers pre-load. A drop in blood pressure is prevented or treated by placing the patient in a supine position or by raising the legs. The most common error with morphine treatment is inadequate dosing. Give 4–8 mg morphine intravenously and follow this with 2–8 mg at 5 to 15 minutes until there is improvement or relief of pain. There will also be improvement in anxiety and restlessness, and a blunting of autonomic output. A rare patient requires large doses of morphine for relief, as much as 2 mg/kg. This is usually tolerated, because patients with cardiac pain or pulmonary edema have a low risk of respiratory depression with morphine. If you are concerned about morphine toxicity as a cause of hypotension,

TABLE 5.4. Beta-Blocker Therapy for Acute MI

Patient selection	Acute MI, <12 hr from the onset of pain
Contraindications	1. Heart failure (rales > 10 cm above the diaphragm) 2. Heart rate < 60 beats/min 3. Heart block (PR > 0.24 sec) 4. Systolic blood pressure < 90 mm Hg 5. Asthma or obstructive lung disease with wheezing
Dosing	**Metoprolol** 5 mg at 5-min intervals for three doses if the heart rate remains > 60/min and the blood pressure > 100 mg Hg Then 100 mg PO qid for 48 hr Then 100 mg PO bid **Atenolol** 5 mg IV infused over 5 min, repeat in 10 min (no second dose if heart rate or blood pressure fall) Then 50 mg PO 10 min later Then 50 mg PO bid
Benefits	Blunts catecholamine effects, lowering heart rate, blood pressure, and contractility. This reduces MVO_2 and thus infarct size. Survival may also be improved by prevention of ventricular fibrillation or LV rupture

severe nausea, or respiratory depression, the effects of morphine are rapidly reversed using naloxone 0.1–0.2 mg intravenously (repeated in 10 to 15 minutes if needed).

β-Adrenergic Blockers

During the acute phase of MI, patients may respond to intravenous beta-blockers with prompt relief of pain and a reduction in ST segment elevation. Randomized trials have shown a reduction in mortality (by 15%), reinfarction (19%), and cardiac arrest (19%). An important mechanism of benefit is reduction of heart rate. The greatest survival benefit is seen during the first day after MI. In contrast, thrombolytic therapy does not reduce mortality during the first 24 hours; a beneficial effect emerges over the next week. Although this suggests a complementary role for beta blockade and reperfusion therapy, synergy has not been supported by clinical trials.

The use of beta-blockers in the acute phase of MI is summarized in Table 5.4. If there is concern about the risk or uncertainty about a contraindication such as a history of bronchospasm, use the short-acting agent esmolol, 50–250 μg/kg/min.

Intravenous Nitroglycerin

When used in the early phase of acute MI, it reduces preload and LV wall tension and therefore myocardial oxygen demand. This

TABLE 5.5. ACE Inhibitor Therapy After Acute MI

Patient selection:
    Strongly indicated: 1, Anterior MI; 2, MI complicated by heart failure; 3, LVEF < 30% after MI
    Uncertain indication: Smaller MI as short-term therapy (clinical trials pending)
Contraindications: Systolic blood pressure < 100 mm Hg, renal artery stenosis, adverse reaction to ACE inhibitors (cough, allergy, rise in creatinine)
Drugs and dose *(start therapy on day 1 of MI)*
    Captopril (Capoten) 12.5–50 mg tid
    Enalapril (Vasotec) 5–20 mg bid
    Lisinopril (Prinivil, Zestril) 2.5–10 mg qd
    Ramipril (Altace) 2.5–5 mg bid
Alternative treatment: Angiotensin II blockers (e.g., losartin), may be substituted for those who cannot tolerate ACE inhibitors

may limit infarct size and prevent infarct expansion. Intravenous nitroglycerin may also dilate collaterals and improve flow to the infarct zone. There have been conflicting results from clinical trials, and the routine use of intravenous nitroglycerin is not established. We do not hesitate to use it when there is ongoing anginal pain. It is safe to use in the face of large infarction and for those with congestive heart failure (when beta blockade may be contraindicated). Nitrates do not depress heart rate or contractility, so they may be used together with beta-blockers; both may depress blood pressure, so monitor carefully.

Early Angiotensin-converting Enzyme Inhibition

Starting angiotensin-converting enzyme (ACE) inhibitors 3 or more days after MI prevents infarct expansion and improves LV function and survival for patients with large MI (Table 5.5). Subsequent trials have found that early treatment—within the first 24 hours—is better for those with large anterior MI. ACE inhibitors may also reduce blood pressure and must be used with caution in patients who have been given intravenous beta-blockers and/or nitroglycerin.

What Drug Should You Choose to Reduce Infarct Size? No drug combination protocol has been studied, and there is no established algorithm. Use of medicines with clear evidence of benefit is sensible (Table 5.6). Addition of other agents will depend on the patient's condition, particularly heart rate and blood pressure. Heart failure and renal dysfunction also influence the choice of drugs.

TABLE 5.6. Treatment to Improve Survival or Limit Infarction Size When Given in the Early Phase of Acute MI

Drug	Evidence for Efficacy	Patients Who Benefit	Contraindications
Coronary thrombolysis	Strong	MI and ST segment elevation or new bundle branch block (See Table 5.7)	See Table 5.8
Aspirin	Strong	All with suspected MI[a]	Allergy or contraindication to aspirin
Intravenous beta-blockers	Strong	All with suspected MI[a], those with tachycardia (see text)	Hypotension, bradycardia, heart block, heart failure, bronchospasm
Intravenous nitroglycerin	Equivocal[b]	Those with anterior MI, ongoing ischemia[a], heart failure	Hypotension, tachycardia, or RV infarction
Oral ACE inhibitors	Strong	Those with anterior MI and ST segment elevation (treat on day 1)	Hypotension, elevated creatinine

[a]If the patient is having unstable angina rather than MI, therapy is still helpful. Beta blockade and nitroglycerin have not been shown to improve survival when given in addition to thrombolytic therapy.
[b]Some, but not all, clinical trials indicate efficacy.

Lidocaine

Prophylactic lidocaine for patients who are in hospital is no longer recommended. Clinical trials found that patients given lidocaine had less VF, but because they were in the coronary care unit (CCU) and had access to DC cardioversion, there was no survival benefit. Separate studies have shown that the incidence of VF during early infarction may be falling, which is further evidence against lidocaine prophylaxis.

There are some clinical settings where prophylactic lidocaine is justified. We use it when CCU monitoring is interrupted. This may include patients being transferred to another hospital during the first 12 hours of MI or those having emergency procedures in the catheterization laboratory. The medicine does work; consider it when defibrillation would be difficult.

The half-life of an initial bolus injection of lidocaine is brief, just minutes. Thus, a bolus must be followed by a continuous infusion. On the other hand, when a patient has been on lidocaine for more than 6 hours and it is then stopped, the half-life is more than 6 hours. For this reason, it makes no sense to "wean" a patient from lidocaine. It is best to stop it first thing in the morning and know that the patient will drift into the subtherapeutic range at mid-day (while you are still in the hospital).

Frequent or complex ventricular premature beats (VPBs > 6/min, multiform VPBs, triplets or R on T VPBs) in the early phase of MI indicate an increased short-term risk of VF and are indications for lidocaine.

Anticoagulation

Full-dose intravenous *heparin* is included in the Practice Guidelines for those with large anterior MI for the prevention of peripheral embolization, and it may be continued to the time of discharge (Table 5.7). If an echocardiogram shows ventricular mural thrombus or a large akinetic segment, *warfarin* should be started before discharge. This anticoagulation regimen may be used for patients with dilated and poorly contracting ventricles as well.

Low-dose heparin (5000 U every 12 hours) may be given to those at bedrest for the prevention of pulmonary embolus. It is usually possible to stop it at 48 hours. For high-risk patients (age > 70, large MI, heart failure, prolonged bedrest, obesity, prior venous disease or pulmonary embolus, physical signs of

TABLE 5.7. Anticoagulation Therapy After MI

Therapy	Indications	Comment
Heparin: short-term, treatment in hospital[a]	Prevention of arterial embolism	Patient selection: 1. Heparin for large, anterior Q-wave MI; continue until discharge. 2. Heparin for those with acute MI, LV dilatation, and low LVEF.
Warfarin: long-term treatment[b]	Prevention of arterial embolism	1. Warfarin after heparin for those with mural thrombus or a dilated akinetic LV apex. Continue for at least 3 months and stop only if the echo shows no thrombus (some advocate indefinite Rx). 2. Indefinite warfarin therapy with LV dilatation and low LVEF or if there is persistent thrombus.
Antiplatelet plus heparin therapy[a]	After reperfusion therapy to prevent early reocclusion	Heparin may be stopped after 2–4 days. Long term therapy with aspirin alone is adequate. After angioplasty or stenting, clopidogrel is frequently added.
Aspirin plus warfarin[b]	Medical treatment of MI without reperfusion therapy	Treatment with warfarin plus aspirin for at least 1 month *may* prevent extension of MI (evidence favors but does not prove efficacy).
Aspirin	Secondary prevention of MI—long-term therapy	Aspirin is the first choice, but clopidogrel or warfarin may be used if there is intolerance to aspirin.[b]
Subcutaneous heparin	Prevention of venous thrombosis and pulmonary embolism early after MI	Heparin 5000 U bid for 2 days. Continue heparin until fully ambulatory if the patient is high risk (age > 70, heart failure, large MI, previous MI, obesity, previous pulmonary embolus or venous disease, prolonged bedrest).
Clopidogrel	Secondary prevention of MI—long-term therapy	A suitable alternative to aspirin, especially when there is aspirin intolerance. In the CAPRI trial, it was superior to aspirin for preventing any ischemic event, but only minimally (risk was lowered 8.7% during the 2-year follow-up), and there has not been a move to this more expensive drug as the first choice.[c] It can also be added to aspirin therapy for the patient with unstable plaque.

This table summarizes practice guidelines (Gunnar RM, Bourdillon PDV, Dixon DW, et al. Guidelines for the early management of patients with acute myocardial infarction. A report of the ACC/AHA Task Force on Assessment of Diagnostic and Therapeutic Cardiovascular Procedures. J Am Coll Cardiol 1990;16:249).

[a]Intravenous heparin to prolong the activated partial thromboplastin time to 1.5–2.0 times control.

[b]Adjust warfarin so that INR = 2.0–3.0.

[c]CAPRI Steering Committee. A randomized blinded trial of clopidogrel versus aspirin in patients at risk of ischaemic events (CAPRIE). Lancet 1996;126:59.

venous insufficiency) it should be continued until they are fully ambulatory.

Calcium Channel Blockers

Most randomized trials found no survival benefit from calcium channel blockade during *transmural (Q wave)* infarction. There was a trend toward increased mortality with nifedipine. In contrast, studies of diltiazem and verapamil showed a trend toward less reinfarction. Nifedipine, a pure vasodilator, causes reflex tachycardia, and the other two drugs depress the sinoatrial node and slow the heart rate. As a rule, drugs that reduce heart rate appear beneficial after MI.

Diltiazem has been shown to reduce the chance of reinfarction for those with *non-Q wave MI.* The Diltiazem Reinfarction Study treated patients with 360 mg diltiazem per day (in four doses) and delayed angiography for 14 days for study purposes. There was less reinfarction and angina in the treated than in the placebo group. There is no reason to delay angiography that long, and this study does not provide a useful treatment model. On the other hand, you will see an occasional patient with non-Q MI who is not a candidate for angiography or revascularization. The study showed that diltiazem treatment may lower the short-term reinfarction risk by 50%. It also identified diltiazem as a useful early therapy while the workup is in progress or when angiography is delayed.

Hemodynamic Monitoring

Severe or progressive heart failure or hypotension and cardiogenic shock are the usual indications for right heart catheterization and hemodynamic monitoring. At times, the cause of hypotension is uncertain, and measurement of LV filling pressure, or preload, distinguishes between LV failure (where it is high) and volume depletion (where it is low). Arterial pressure monitoring may be used to monitor patients on vasopressor therapy and those with hypotension.

Right heart catheterization is also useful when managing rupture of the interventricular septum or acute papillary muscle dysfunction and mitral regurgitation.

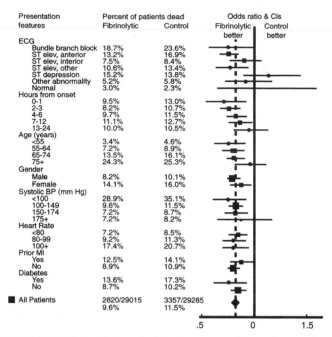

Presentation features	Percent of patients dead		Odds ratio & CIs	
	Fibrinolytic	Control	Fibrinolytic better	Control better
ECG				
Bundle branch block	18.7%	23.6%		
ST elev, anterior	13.2%	16.9%		
ST elev, interior	7.5%	8.4%		
ST elev, other	10.6%	13.4%		
ST depression	15.2%	13.8%		
Other abnormality	5.2%	5.8%		
Normal	3.0%	2.3%		
Hours from onset				
0-1	9.5%	13.0%		
2-3	8.2%	10.7%		
4-6	9.7%	11.5%		
7-12	11.1%	12.7%		
13-24	10.0%	10.5%		
Age (years)				
<55	3.4%	4.6%		
55-64	7.2%	8.9%		
65-74	13.5%	16.1%		
75+	24.3%	25.3%		
Gender				
Male	8.2%	10.1%		
Female	14.1%	16.0%		
Systolic BP (mm Hg)				
<100	28.9%	35.1%		
100-149	9.6%	11.5%		
150-174	7.2%	8.7%		
175+	7.2%	8.2%		
Heart Rate				
<80	7.2%	8.5%		
80-99	9.2%	11.3%		
100+	17.4%	20.7%		
Prior MI				
Yes	12.5%	14.1%		
No	8.9%	10.9%		
Diabetes				
Yes	13.6%	17.3%		
No	8.7%	10.2%		
■ All Patients	2820/29015	3357/29285		
	9.6%	11.5%		

FIGURE 5.6. Effects of thrombolytic therapy on 1-month mortality after acute MI. Pooled data from nine placebo controlled trials, including 58,600 patients. (From the Fibrinolytic Therapy Trialists' Collaborative Group. Lancet 1994;343:311.)

THROMBOLYTIC THERAPY FOR ACUTE MI____

Reperfusion therapy is the standard of care for MI with ST segment elevation. You must be able to use it if you treat patients with acute MI. Chest pain usually begins within 5 minutes of coronary artery occlusion, and myocardial cell death is progressive beyond that point. With each quarter hour that passes, more heart muscle is lost. Early reperfusion saves more lives than later reperfusion (Fig. 5.6). The patient in the emergency room does not have time to wait for a cardiologist to arrive and make a decision. The first doctor to see the patient in the emergency room should initiate treatment.

Pathophysiology of Reperfusion

Randomized clinical trials have shown that the benefits of early reperfusion exceed negative effects, but there are potential problems. "Reperfusion injury" is possible but is of uncertain clinical significance. Animal studies have shown that transient coronary occlusion followed by abrupt reperfusion leads to additional myocardial injury (with a histologic pattern called "contraction band necrosis"). Early angiography in patients occasionally shows a "no reflow" phenomenon, or poor distal flow and runoff despite an open coronary artery. This has been attributed to microvascular damage. In addition, injured vessels are leaky, leading to hemorrhagic infarction, although the region of hemorrhagic infarct has not been shown to extend beyond the area of necrosis. Finally, there may be loss of coronary vasodilator reserve with injury of small vessels. These complications of reperfusion may contribute to *stunned myocardium*, temporary contractile dysfunction after reperfusion that may take weeks to improve.

Reperfusion arrhythmias, an "electrical storm," often develop with restoration of flow. Accelerated idioventricular ventricular rhythm (AIVR), also called "slow ventricular tachycardia (VT)," is so common that it has been suggested as a marker of reperfusion. It is generally benign and tends not to degenerate to VF. The mechanism of AIVR is discharge from an automatic focus. VF is caused by reentry, a different mechanism. AIVR often is treated with lidocaine, but it tends not to respond.

Although it is possible for VF to occur with reperfusion, it is unusual, and prophylactic lidocaine is not recommended. A review of large trials found that the risk of VF is not increased by thrombolytic therapy.

Patients with inferior MI may develop bradyarrhythmias with reperfusion, possibly due to the Bezold-Jarish reflex. These are usually transient and do not require pacemaker therapy.

Illusion of Reperfusion and Early Reocclusion

An angiogram showing an open infarct artery soon after thrombolytic therapy suggests but does not prove a benefit to the patient. No reflow, mentioned above, is a possible mechanism. On the angiogram there is slow washout of contrast from the artery and infarct zone.

Other patients snatch defeat from the jaws of victory by reoccluding the open infarct artery, usually without recurrence of chest pain. Reocclusion of an initially patent infarct artery was reported in 29% of patients in one trial who had repeat angiography

3 months later. Only 20% of them had chest pain with reocclusion. Those with silent reocclusion had a worse clinical course. *Silent ischemia* after thrombolysis is common, because transient ischemia followed by reperfusion stuns cardiac pain receptors, just as it does myocardium.

Indications for Thrombolytic Therapy

The basis for patient selection for any treatment is weighing benefits and risks: Doctors and their patients must play the odds. MI often is fatal, justifying the use of high-risk therapy.

The chance of dying from some heart attacks is higher than with others. As noted in Figure 5.6, clinical trials have shown that thrombolytic therapy improves survival for those with higher but not lower risk infarction. In fact, patients with chest pain and suspected MI but without ECG changes had an increase in mortality with thrombolytic therapy.

Patient selection is not as simple as just interpreting the ECG. Multiple other clinical features raise mortality during MI, including advanced age, heart failure, female sex, diabetes, and a history of prior infarction. Table 5.8 suggests a hierarchy of MI risk and identifies clinical features influential in favor of reperfusion therapy for the patient with a borderline ECG indication.

Specific Patient Selection Issues
Inferior MI

Many patients having a first infarction have an inferior MI. As infarction of the inferior wall tends to injure less muscle than anterior MI, the short-term mortality risk is much lower. With low mortality it is difficult to show a survival benefit with reperfusion therapy. Clinical trials demonstrating improved survival with reperfusion did not stratify those with inferior MI into high- and low-risk groups, and it is probable that a survival benefit was limited to higher risk patients.

Recall that these studies examined short-term mortality. When considering long-term survival, any salvage of muscle may be important. For this reason, I am biased in favor of treating a young person with a small inferior MI when it is possible to treat early. If therapy is to be applied late in the course of MI, more

TABLE 5.8. Patient Selection for Reperfusion Therapy Based on the Risk of Death from MI

Hierarchy of MI Risk	Other Clinical Features that Increase the Risk of MI and thus Weigh in Favor of Reperfusion Therapy
Highest risk, definitely treat:	Heart Failure
Anterior MI with ST elevation	History of heart failure
Large Inferior MI[a]	Rales (Killip class II)
Acute MI with new bundle branch block	Pulmonary edema (Killip class III)
	Cardiogenic shock (Killip class IV)
Lower risk, consider reperfusion therapy based on	History of prior MI (more likely to have low LVEF)
other clinical features:	Right ventricular infarct syndrome
Small inferior MI with ST elevation[a]	Diabetes
MI with ST depression or T wave inversion and pain unresponsive to conventional therapy[b]	

[a]*Large inferior MI:* marked (as opposed to minimal) ST elevation in inferior leads plus reciprocal ST depression in anterior or lateral leads or ST elevation in right precordial leads indicating the RV infarction syndrome.
Small inferior MI: minimal ST elevation in inferior leads, no reciprocal ST depression.
[b]Including nitrates, chewed aspirin, heparin, and beta-blockers.

159

than 4 hours after the onset of pain, the risks of thrombolytic therapy for a low-risk MI may exceed benefits.

Inferior MI and Hypotension

Acute inferior MI is often accompanied by vagal discharge, which causes bradycardia, nausea, and hypotension. This responds to intravenous fluid replacement (normal saline is my first choice) and atropine if the heart rate is low. A vagal reaction during inferior MI does not contraindicate thrombolytic therapy.

Hypotension may also indicate RV failure secondary to RV infarction. The mortality rate with this form of cardiogenic shock is above 30%. RV infarction is complicated by high degree atrioventricular (AV) block in about half the patients. Other complications of MI also are more common, including ventricular septal rupture, RV thrombus, and pulmonary embolus. Interestingly, most with RV infarction also have significant LV dysfunction. RV infarction has not been the subject of randomized trials because of small numbers of patients, but there is a consensus that early reperfusion therapy is indicated.

Acute MI Without ST Segment Elevation and Unstable Angina

Studies of reperfusion therapy for non-Q wave MI have shown no survival benefit (Fig. 5.6). This comes as no surprise, because clinical experience has taught us that there is usually prompt resolution of chest discomfort with aggressive antianginal therapy (nitrates, aspirin, beta blockade, and heparin). Angiography during the acute phase of non-Q infarction and in those with unstable angina usually shows a patent, though tightly stenosed, infarct artery. Thrombolytic therapy is not required to restore flow.

If a patient with symmetric T wave inversion and/or ST depression continues to have pain after initial treatment, our first step is to reconsider the diagnosis. If the ST and T wave changes are new and we are convinced that myocardial ischemia is responsible for the pain, we would consider thrombolysis or angioplasty. When there is uncertainty about the diagnosis, angiography and possible angioplasty would be safer than thrombolytic therapy.

Ischemic Chest Pain and No ECG Changes

Lateral MI may not cause ST segment deviation. For this reason, a normal ECG does not exclude MI. Fortunately, the lateral infarctions that present in this manner are small and therefore low risk. It is doubtful that thrombolytic therapy would favorably influence mortality, and it is not indicated.

Consider other diagnoses when there are no ECG changes. Severe chest discomfort with diaphoresis may also be caused by aortic dissection or esophageal rupture, illnesses where thrombolysis could be disastrous.

There is one other thing to remember in this situation: *Repeat the ECG.* It is common for patients with subtle or no ECG changes to have clearcut ST elevation on a repeat ECG 15 to 30 minutes later, especially if pain worsens.

Advanced Age

Although age above 65 years increases mortality with acute MI, I do not include advanced age as a factor that weighs in favor of thrombolytic therapy (Table 5.8). The reason for this is that elderly people also have an increased risk of hemorrhagic stroke after thrombolysis. The risk of stroke for those in the GUSTO-I trial for those less than 65 years old was 0.8%, between 65 and 74 years, 2.1%, and between 75 and 85 years, 3.4%. The chance of other bleeding complications is higher as well.

An increased risk of stroke does not mandate avoiding thrombolytic therapy. But it does require careful evaluation for contraindications to therapy (vide infra). In community practice, most of the elderly patients who are treated are healthy and active. Few doctors use this aggressive treatment strategy for debilitated patients from the nursing home.

Chest Pain Has Resolved But ST Segment Elevation Persists

Symptoms may wax and wane during the initial stage of MI. During the intracoronary STK era we were able to observe the coronary artery in the catheterization laboratory while monitoring symptoms and the ECG. We often saw arteries open and then reocclude. Many patients did not have a return of pain with reocclusion, despite reelevation of ST segments. In a sense, the patient developed silent ischemia, possibly because of stunned pain receptors. If the patient is within 6 hours of the onset of MI and still has ST elevation, proceed with thrombolytic therapy. On the other hand, if the patient has had chest pain all night, it resolves the next day, and the ST segements are still elevated, we would be less inclined to treat. This sounds more like a completed MI.

Persistent Chest Pain and ST Elevation, But Q Waves Have Evolved

There is a misconception that Q waves always indicate completed injury. With reperfusion, and even with transient reperfusion, Q waves may develop in minutes. It is not unusual to see Q waves soon after the onset of MI, early enough in the course of infarction that there is still viable muscle. Q waves do not contraindicate thrombolytic therapy, nor do they indicate that it is too late to save muscle.

Late Treatment

Clinical trials showed no benefit when thrombolysis is given more than 12 hours after the onset of MI (Fig. 5.6). The LATE study specifically addressed this issue and showed a small benefit when recombinant tissue plasminogen activator (rt-PA) was given between 6 and 12 hours after the onset of symptoms, but not after 12 hours.

An important clinical issue is the potential increase in *myocardial rupture* with late thrombolysis (≥12 hours from the onset). Other complications of thrombolysis occur with similar frequency in patients treated early and late.

In clinical practice I avoid thrombolytic therapy for those having lower risk MI unless it can be given within 6 hours of the onset. In the presence of higher risk infarction, I do not hesitate to treat as late as 12 hours. Beyond 12 hours I occasionally treat a patient with continued pain and ST elevation who is having a high-risk MI and who is at low risk for complications. It is a judgment call; carefully explain not only risks and benefits but also the fact that the indication for therapy is marginal. If possible, consider angioplasty rather than thrombolysis for late reperfusion because of the chance of myocardial rupture.

TABLE 5.9. Contraindications to Thrombolytic Therapy

Absolute contraindications
  Active internal bleeding
  History of cerebrovascular accident
  Recent (within 2 mo) intracranial or intraspinal surgery or trauma
  Intracranial neoplasm, arteriovenous malformation, or aneurysm
  Known bleeding diathesis
  Severe uncontrolled hypertension

Relative contraindications
  Recent (within 10 days) major surgery, e.g., coronary artery bypass graft,
    obstetric delivery, organ biopsy, previous puncture of noncompressible
    vessels
  Cerebrovascular disease
  Recent gastrointestinal or genitourinary bleeding (within 10 days)
  Recent trauma (within 10 days)
  Hypertension: systolic BP ≥180 mm Hg and/or diastolic BP ≥110 mm Hg
  High likelihood of left heart thrombus, e.g., mitral stenosis with atrial
    fibrillation
  Acute pericarditis
  Subacute bacterial endocarditis
  Hemostatic defects including those resulting from severe hepatic or renal
    disease
  Significant liver dysfunction
  Pregnancy
  Diabetic hemorrhagic retinopathy or other hemorrhagic ophthalmic
    conditions
  Septic thrombophlebitis or occluded atrioventricular cannula at seriously
    infected site
  Advanced age, i.e., over 75 yr
  Patients currently receiving oral anticoagulants, e.g., warfarin
  Any other condition in which bleeding constitutes a significant hazard or
    would be particularly difficult to manage because of its location

Syndromes mimicking MI that carry a high risk of bleeding
  Peptic esophagitis
  Pericarditis
  Aortic dissection
  Intracranial bleeding with T wave changes

Contraindications to Thrombolytic Therapy
(Table 5.9)

The most important patient selection issue is the risk of bleeding. Risk is relative. A patient with a high-risk MI and a relative contraindication possibly should have thrombolysis, whereas another having a small first infarction should not. Most bleeding is minor, occurring at vascular puncture sites. As a rule it can be controlled with local pressure.

Intracranial hemorrhage is the worst complication, with an incidence of 0.75% in the large clinical trials. When the usual contraindications to therapy are followed, especially a history of prior stroke, an individual's chance of hemorrhagic stroke increases with any of four different risk factors: age more than 65 years, weight less than 70 kg, hypertension on presentation (systolic pressure ≥ 170 mm Hg or diastolic pressure ≥ 95 mm Hg), and use of rt-PA rather than STK. The probability of bleeding was related to the number of these risk factors: 0.26% with none, 0.96% with one, 1.32% with two, and 2.17% with three. Note that these clinical trials excluded patients with contraindications, including "uncontrolled hypertension," which most studies defined as sustained systolic pressure greater than 200 mm Hg or diastolic pressure less than 110 mm Hg. If you mistakenly treat patients with prior stroke or uncontrolled hypertension, a higher incidence of intracranial hemorrhage may be expected.

Relative Contraindications to Thrombolytic Therapy
Invasive Procedures

Recent surgery and percutaneous biopsy of lung, pleura, liver, or kidneys are strong contraindications to thrombolysis. If less than 2 weeks from the procedure, count on bleeding. At 3 to 6 weeks postprocedure the risk of bleeding still is high, and the decision to use thrombolytic therapy should be related to the risk of the MI. Would you consider thrombolysis in a patient with recent cardiac catheterization? Possibly, because bleeding from the groin can be controlled with local pressure, and the ability to control bleeding enters into the assessment of risk. Angioplasty as therapy for MI would be preferable for those with an excessive bleeding risk.

Coagulation Disorders

The risk of bleeding appears related to the severity of the underlying disorder. A prior history of bleeding indicates higher risk. A borderline low platelet count is not a contraindication to thrombolysis. Some hospitals make the mistake of requiring coagulation studies before starting thrombolytic therapy. In the absence of a history of bleeding diathesis, waiting for these laboratory results unnecessarily delays treatment of the MI.

Cardiopulmonary Resuscitation

Patients with acute MI who have VF and brief periods of cardiopulmonary resuscitation can be treated with thrombolytic agents with reasonable safety. On the other hand, when cardiopulmonary resuscitation is prolonged beyond 10 minutes or when there is obvious chest wall trauma during resuscitation or intubation, the bleeding risk increases. (Again, weigh the risk of the MI.) Thrombolytic therapy should not be given as a part of a prolonged resuscitation attempt.

Diabetic Retinopathy

Our ophthalmology colleagues believe that there is an increased risk of intraocular bleeding with thrombolysis, although the complication has not been mentioned even by the larger studies. Retinopathy remains a relative contraindication, and I would recommend thrombolysis only for those with high-risk MI.

Menstruation and Pregnancy

I have treated a few patients in their 40s during menstruation, and excessive bleeding has not been a problem. Bleeding may improve with hormonal therapy, which could be considered for the menstruating patient with a high-risk MI. Avoid thrombolysis during pregnancy or within 1-month postpartum. Angioplasty is safer.

Anticoagulation or Prior Thrombolytic Therapy

Warfarin therapy does not contraindicate coronary thrombolysis for those with high-risk MI. It would be one reason to avoid it for low-risk infarction. Aspirin is not a contraindication. Prior treatment with STK leads to antibody formation, and such patients should be treated with rt-PA (which is not antigenic).

Pharmacology of Thrombolytic Therapy

Damage to plaque surface exposes collagen that, in turn, activates platelets and leads to the formation of a platelet plug. This also triggers the clotting cascade whose end product is thrombin, a protease that mediates conversion of fibrinogen to fibrin. Fibrin is bound to the platelet plug and is the insoluble, noncellular, fibrous component of thrombus. This is a natural process that allows repair of vascular injury. But it is also the pathologic process that leads to formation of occlusive thrombus on the surface of ulcerated plaque.

Clot formation and dissolution are in dynamic equilibrium. Developing thrombus cannot be allowed to propagate indefinitely, and clot within blood vessels or in ureters must eventually be removed to restore patency. This is the role of the thrombolytic, or fibrinolytic, system. As soon as thrombus forms, the fibrinolytic system is activated.

Plasminogen is the precursor of the active fibrinolytic enzyme, plasmin (Fig. 5.7). Plasminogen is converted to plasmin by "plasminogen activators." These include the naturally occurring substances, t-PA and urokinase, and the foreign compound, STK.

Plasminogen is produced by the liver and is found in the circulation. When clot forms, this free plasminogen is incorporated into the thrombus and is bound to fibrin. The ideal thrombolytic agent would move into the thrombus and work only on fibrin-bound plasminogen. But most of the thrombolytic agents activate free circulating plasminogen as well, producing plasmin and the so-called lytic state (Fig. 5.7). Free plasmin digests circulating fibrinogen and other clotting factors, producing an hypocoagulable state.

Thrombolytic Drug Preparations

STK works on both circulating and fibrin-bound plasminogen and thus produces a lytic state. After STK treatment, there is marked depletion of fibrinogen levels. Because it is a foreign compound, STK is antigenic, and allergic reactions occur in about 2%. It should not be used when there is a history of STK administration during the previous year. Transient hypotension develops in 10%, responding to recumbence or elevation of the legs. This vasodilator response is not an allergic reaction.

Urokinase is a protein found in urine. It has less fibrin affinity than other agents, and uptake into thrombus is limited. It thus induces a systemic lytic state, and relies upon the circulating plasmin that is formed to digest thrombus. It is no more effective than STK in opening occluded coronary arteries, and there have been no clinical trials establishing a survival benefit. It is not approved for intravenous treatment of acute MI.

t-PA, either native or recombinant, works primarily at the tissue level on fibrin-bound plasminogen, so there is less depletion of circulating fibrinogen. It relies upon fibrin as a cofactor, and when bound to fibrin, its activity in cleaving (activating) plasminogen is increased 500-fold. That is why it is referred to as a clot-specific, or "tissue level," plasminogen activator. When not bound to fibrin and free in the circulation, it is not as potent.

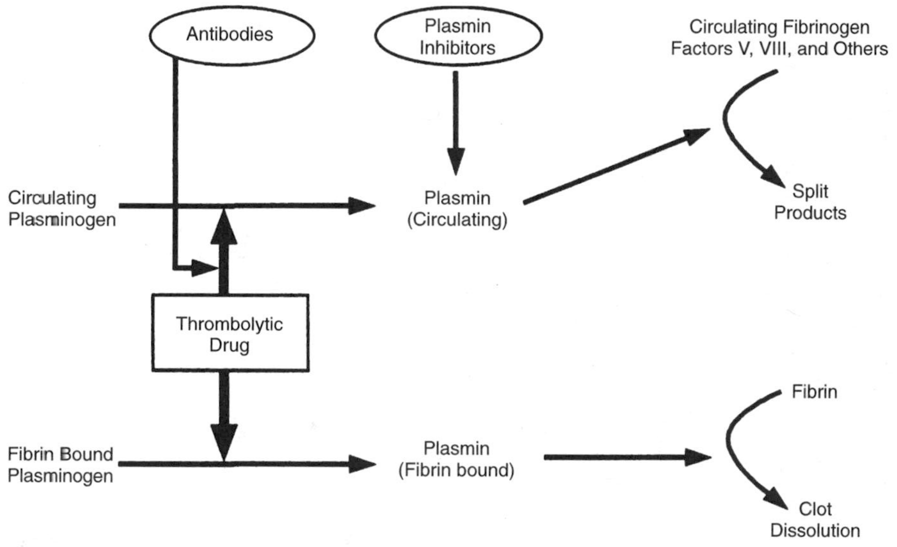

FIGURE 5.7. Sites of action of thrombolytic drugs. Ideally, the drug moves into the thrombus and activates fibrin-bound plasminogen, leading to prompt clot dissolution. In varying degrees, and depending on tissue affinity, thrombolytics also work on circulating plasminogen, producing free plasmin. Free plasmin may also dissolve clot, but it also lyses circulating fibrinogen and other clotting factors. High levels of free plasmin and low levels of circulating fibrinogen constitute the "lytic state." Plasmin inhibitors may neutralize circulating plasmin, and antibodies may neutralize streptokinase. (Reproduced by permission from Taylor GJ. Thrombolytic Therapy for Acute Myocardial Infarction. Cambridge, MA: Blackwell Science, 1992.)

There is usually some depletion of fibrinogen during rt-PA treatment, as the dose of rt-PA is much greater than circulating levels of native t-PA. But patients are not as hypocoagulable as they are after STK therapy. For this reason anticoagulation is necessary after infusion of rt-PA.

There are two available forms of t-PA: recombinant t-PA (alteplase) and its mutant form, reteplase. The altered structure of reteplase results in slower clearance, so that it can be given as a bolus rather than a continuous intravenous infusion.

Choice of Agent

The GUSTO-1 study (the mother of all clinical trials with 41,021 patients) showed that rt-PA (alteplase) is more effective than STK when front-loaded dosing is used. The reason for the 14.6% reduction in 30-day mortality with rt-PA is probably explained by more rapid and complete thrombolysis. Angiography 90 minutes after starting therapy showed a higher rate of TIMI grade 3 (brisk) flow in the rt-PA group. The newer rt-PA preparation, reteplace, has efficacy and risks similar to alteplase. It may be given as two intravenous bolus injections, and our nurses prefer this convenience to the 90-minute infusion of alteplase. The cost of the two drugs is similar.

An often discussed drug selection issue is the increase in hemorrhagic stroke with rt-PA, raising the possibility that elderly patients who have a higher risk of stroke should be treated with STK (see the earlier discussion of older patients). A careful analysis of the data indicates that for patients less than 85 years old, rt-PA treatment is better than STK in lowering the combined rate of death and disabling stroke (there are a few more strokes, but many fewer deaths, for a net clinical benefit). An elderly patient with a large anterior MI who can be treated early, especially within 1 to 2 hours from the onset of symptoms, would clearly benefit from more rapid thrombolysis with rt-PA. On the other hand, if therapy is begun more than 4 hours from the onset of MI, there is less muscle salvage, and the benefits of thrombolysis may be limited to other effects of an open infarct artery. Speed of thrombolysis is less critical with late therapy, and STK would be a reasonable choice, especially when the risk of stroke is higher than usual. Tailoring thrombolytic therapy to the risk of the MI, the risk of complications, and the timing of treatment applies to younger patients as well.

A practical note: The nuances of drug selection may elude you in the middle of the night when dealing with an acutely ill patient. *When in doubt, you cannot go wrong using one of the rt-PA preparations.*

Management after Thrombolysis
Antiplatelet Therapy

The ISIS-2 trial established that *chewed aspirin* at the time of presentation increases survival for those treated with STK (Fig. 5.5). Platelet inhibition has a number of beneficial effects. First, thrombolytic drugs work on fibrin, and there is little fibrin in the fresh clot. This platelet-rich thrombus is relatively resistant to fibrinolytic therapy, because aggregated platelets secrete PAI-1, which blocks fibrinolysis (Fig. 5.7). Second, when fibrin is lysed, there is exposure of thrombin. Thrombin is a potent activator of platelets, so fibrinolysis has the paradoxical procoagulant effect of promoting platelet aggregation.

It is interesting that even the weak antiplatelet action of aspirin improved outcome in ISIS-2. Trials of more effective anti-platelet therapy using glycoprotein IIb/IIIa blockers with lower dose rt-PA (to minimize its procoagulant effect) are finding an even more rapid and complete restoration of coronary flow, and this will probably be the treatment of choice.

Antithrombotic Therapy

Those treated with t-PA preparations have little fibrinogen deple-tion and are not anticoagulated. Heparin therapy is used after treatment with rt-PA, and the activated partial thromboplastin time should be in the therapeutic range, 1.5 to 2 times control. It is common for the activated partial thromboplastin time to be longer during the first 24 hours. Do not interrupt heparin ther-apy or reduce the dose. Instead, recheck the activated partial thromboplastin time at 24 hours and adjust the dose. The more potent antithrombin agents, hirudin and hirulog, are no more effective than heparin in this setting.

Other Medical Therapy

The TIMI-2 trial evaluated intravenous metoprolol as an adjunct to coronary thrombolysis and found no effect on survival or LV function. There was a reduction in recurrent ischemia and reinfarction. We use beta blockade for those with sinus tachycardia and/or hypertension when there is no evidence of heart failure.

Calcium channel blockers, intravenous nitroglycerin, ACE inhibitors, and intravenous magnesium have been proposed as treatment that may reduce infarct size. None has been shown to augment the benefits of reperfusion therapy.

Assessment of Reperfusion and Prognosis

Coronary angiography is the gold standard for identifying an open infarct artery after thrombolytic therapy. Relief of pain, when dramatic, is a fair marker of reperfusion. However, many with an open artery and myocardial salvage continue to have some discomfort, and there is often uncertainty based on symptoms. Reperfusion arrhythmias have not proved reliable markers either. With reperfusion, there is rapid washout of CK-MB and other enzymes from the infarct zone, and this combined with relief of chest discomfort and reduction in ST segment elevation provides the best noninvasive index of reperfusion.

Early improvement in ST segment elevation indicates a better prognosis after thrombolysis. Patients with continued elevation or just minimal reduction in ST elevation are more likely to have persistent occlusion with the expected clinical consequences: worse LV function, increased morbidity, and higher short- and long-term mortality. Thus, repeating the ECG at 1 and 3 hours after starting thrombolytic therapy is useful for estimating prognosis.

Angiography and Revascularization

Ideally, angiography would be recommended for patients with successful thrombolysis and salvage of myocardium who are at high risk for reocclusion. Others could be treated medically. Some treatment failures are obvious: late application, no resolution of pain or ST elevation, and slow washout of CK-MB (or another of the cardiac enzymes). When this is clearcut, medical therapy to optimize LV function and reduce morbidity would be reasonable.

For most patients there is uncertainty about the status of the infarct artery after thrombolytic therapy. Exercise testing may be misleading; one study reported that ST depression with exercise was more common with an occluded than with an open infarct artery. Nor does perfusion imaging reliably identify the patient with a poor prognosis. Because of uncertainty, the trend in clinical practice has been angiography for most after coronary thrombolysis, especially when there are clinical indicators of reperfusion. The balance of data favors revascularization when the infarct artery is tightly stenosed.

PRIMARY ANGIOPLASTY FOR ACUTE MI_____

Angioplasty is an effective method for opening the infarct artery, and it works faster than thrombolytic therapy. Patients who come to our emergency room with acute MI have at least a 90% chance of having an open infarct artery within 60 minutes if they can be taken directly to the catheterization laboratory. No study of thrombolytic drug therapy matches that result, and it is the approach that we take whenever possible.

The problem, of course, is logistical. Accomplishing the goal—an open artery within 60 minutes—requires an open catheterization laboratory and a qualified team that is ready for the patient. Most programs are not organized to provide 24-hour or weekend service. Most important, only some patients are initially treated in hospitals with angioplasty services. The time required to transfer the patient removes the major advantage of the procedure, speed.

Most now agree with angioplasty when it can be done quickly by an experienced team, and that has been incorporated into the newest Practice Guidelines. On the other hand, the results with angioplasty are not compelling enough to warrant delay of treatment or to justify cross-country transfer for a midnight balloon. Nor are they compelling enough that we must install catheterization laboratories at major crossroads. Despite enthusiasm for this technique, I expect that most patients with acute MI in the United States will be properly treated in the emergency rooms of community hospitals using coronary thrombolysis. Regardless of your approach, the emphasis in your practice should be on rapid treatment.

COMPLICATIONS OF MI_____

Cardiogenic Shock
Before the reperfusion era, cardiogenic shock developed in about 20% of patients with MI, and the mortality rate was as high as

80% (Table 5.2, from the classic study of Killip and Kimble). With modern therapy, the incidence has fallen to 7% and the mortality rate to about 40%. Nevertheless, LV failure and cardiogenic shock remain the leading cause of in-hospital death with MI.

Pathophysiology

In 80% of cases, shock is caused by excessive damage to the left ventricle. Autopsy studies have shown that the pump loses its ability to maintain blood pressure when 40% of the left ventricle is infarcted. The remaining cases result from other mechanical complications of MI (Table 5.10). It is important to recognize these quickly, because the treatment approach may be different.

When LV injury, or pump failure, is the cause of shock, there is a series of potentially harmful compensatory responses. An increase in sympathethic tone and activation of the renin-angiotensin system both raise peripheral vascular resistance and ventricular afterload, further depressing LV function. The drop in arterial pressure lowers coronary perfusion pressure, aggravating ischemia. Unfortunately, most patients with cardiogenic shock have multivessel disease. Collateral vessels may be supplied by a stenosed artery, which magnifies the effect of lower perfusion pressure. It is the worst of all possible worlds: decreasing coronary flow, further ischemic injury, and depression of LV function in a progressive, stuttering fashion.

Shock is present in only 10% of patients at the time of hospital admission and develops in the remaining 90% during the first day or two. Loss of muscle at the edge of the infarct zone may have a role in the genesis of LV failure. Muscle in this watershed zone is dependent on collateral flow and may be viable (and salvageable) in the early hours of infarction; with low perfusion pressure it becomes a late casualty. Prolonged elevation of CK-MB may reflect a stuttering pattern of injury.

Clinical Presentation

The hemodynamic definition of cardiogenic shock includes persistent hypotension with systolic arterial pressure < 80 mm Hg, low cardiac index (cardiac output corrected for body surface area < 1.8 L/min/m^2), and elevated LV filling pressure (pulmonary wedge pressure > 18 mm Hg).

TABLE 5.10. Pathophysiology of Heart Failure or Cardiogenic Shock after Acute MI

Mechanism	Clinical and Laboratory Findings	Hemodynamic Findings
LV failure (the most common cause of cardiogenic shock)	Most common with anterior MI; possible history or ECG evidence of prior MI; usually pulmonary congestion; Echo = low LVEF and extensive wall motion abnormalities.	Elevated LV filling pressure (pulmonary wedge pressure), low cardiac output (CO), hypotension.
RV infarction	Inferior MI, pulmonary congestion usually not present; jugular venous distention and edema following hydration; pulsus paradoxus; ST elevation in right precordial leads (V_{4R}); Echo = RV dilatation and hypokinesis, possibly normal LV function and a small left ventricle.	Elevated right atrial and RV diastolic pressure, low or normal LV filling pressure (though it may be high if there is associated LV failure), low CO.
Acute mitral regurgitation (MR)	Murmur of MR (but it may be soft), severe pulmonary congestion; Echo = MR on the Doppler study; possibly a flail mitral leaflet. LV function may be only minimally depressed.	Elevated LV filling pressure and tall V wave on the pulmonary wedge tracing, low CO.
Ventricular septal defect (VSD)	Inferior or anterior MI, systolic murmur (may be soft or absent), often pulmonary congestion; Echo = left to right shunt on the Doppler study, and no MR. LV function may not be depressed.	Elevated LV filling pressure, but no V wave; "step-up" in O_2 saturation documents the shunt (saturation in the pulmonary artery is higher than mixed venous O_2 saturation)
Rupture of the ventricular free wall	Often a small first MI (see text for clinical profile). Usually sudden death, with no time for an echo. Cardiac tamponade.	Findings of cardiac tamponade, but rarely time for catheterization.

173

Most patients with shock and elevated LV filling pressure also have severe pulmonary congestion. The diagnosis is fairly certain when there is low blood pressure, pulmonary edema, and clinical evidence of poor perfusion (cool clammy skin, low urine output, and altered sensorium).

Those with shock in a setting of first MI are usually having a large anterior MI. A small infarction may cause LV failure when there has been prior infarction or heart failure; remember that LV injury is cumulative. Shock is more common in older patients and those with multivessel CAD, and both indicate a worse prognosis.

Management of Cardiogenic Shock

Laboratory Evaluation The clinical findings suggest the diagnosis. Hemodynamic measurements confirm it, and monitoring helps with adjustment of inotropic support. An echocardiogram at the bedside shows severe LV dysfunction and excludes other conditions. If your hospital does not routinely use pulmonary artery catheterization in its intensive care unit, an echocardiogram would be the next best diagnostic study. The ECG usually confirms a large MI.

Treatment Supportive care of patients with shock is aimed at maintaining blood pressure and end-organ perfusion. The goal is to raise coronary perfusion pressure and stop the cycle of continued ischemia and LV injury. When there is hypotension but no pulmonary congestion, a fluid challenge is a good initial maneuver. Give 200 mL normal saline quickly, intravenously, and repeat it at 30-minute intervals. Carefully monitor the chest examination during fluid loading, and stop if there is any evidence for congestion.

Catecholamine therapy is usually needed to treat hypotension due to LV failure, but it does not improve survival. Indeed, catechols increase myocardial oxygen demand and may aggravate ischemia. Consider pharmacologic support of blood pressure and cardiac output a temporizing measure. The preferred agents are dobutamine, a pure inotropic agent with few noncardiac effects and low arrhythmogenic potential, and dopamine, which is also a renal vasodilator that promotes diuresis. At high doses, above 10 µg/kg/min, the selective actions of these drugs disappear; they work as pure vasoconstrictors, and LV filling pressure rises. Combining dopamine and dobutamine is useful. When each is given at rates as high as 7.5 µg/kg/min, cardiac output and blood pressure rise without an increase in LV filling pressure.

Intraaortic balloon pump (IABP) counterpulsation raises blood pressure, lowers afterload, and improves cardiac output and therefore coronary and coronary collateral perfusion pressure. At the same time, it reduces the workload of the heart. Of all possible supportive therapies, it is the most effective. But without revascularizaiton, the IABP does not improve survival. The classic study of IABP treatment alone from the early 1970s showed a short-term hemodynamic benefit but 83% in-hospital and 91% 1-year mortality. Many of these patients became "balloon dependent"; they were fine while the pump was working but slipped back into shock when it was turned off. Getting stuck on the pump is a risk of using IABP support when there is no hope of reversing the shock syndrome with revascularization.

Coronary thrombolysis, alone, may not be enough to save the patient. Early placebo controlled trials had few patients who were in shock at the time of thrombolytic therapy, and some of them found no benefit. Reperfusion may be more difficult to achieve when pressure is low. Even with an open artery, low perfusion pressure may not allow excellent (TIMI grade 3) flow. Nevertheless, there is a general belief that a fast-acting thrombolytic agent, one of the rt-PA preparations, may help patients in shock when given early, within 3 to 4 hours of the onset of MI. Late therapy does not help once shock is established.

On the other hand, it is well established that reperfusion therapy *prevents* shock. The incidence of shock was reduced by about 50% in placebo controlled studies. The GUSTO-1 trial found less shock and heart failure with rt-PA, which opens arteries faster than STK.

Early revascularization may be the key to successful treatment. The SHOCK trial found no survival benefit at 30 days but a significant one at 6 months. Subgroup analysis showed that benefit was limited to patients less than 75 years old. Older patients had increased mortality with revascularization. The 30-day mortality of younger patients was 41% with angioplasty versus 57% with medical therapy (this is a bad disease).

For revascularization to work, it must be accomplished early. The day after MI is no good. If fact, the odds are against angioplasty helping when a patient has been in shock more than 10 hours. You must achieve reperfusion within 6 hours of the onset of MI, and preferably within 4 hours.

The best treatment strategy: As soon as you make a clinical diagnosis of cardiogenic shock and agree with the patient and family that aggressive treatment is the correct approach, begin moving the patient to the catheterization laboratory. Do this even if the patient has received thrombolytic therapy. Second, initiate supportive measures to raise blood pressure to 80 to 90 mm Hg. Third, in the catheterization laboratory a few things are done; the diagnosis is confirmed, an IABP is inserted, and angiography and angioplasty are performed. The IABP is particularly helpful, because it raises coronary perfusion pressure and prevents reocclusion of the dilated artery. It usually can be removed within a couple of days.

If your hospital does not have revascularization capabilities, shock is an indication for emergency transfer. Do not take the patient to the coronary care unit with plans to try medical therapy, a Swan-Ganz catheter, and so forth unless you have made the decision to avoid revascularization. It is a waste of time.

Right Ventricular (RV) Infarct Syndrome

The RV infarct syndrome is a cause of shock that may complicate inferior MI. About one half of all patients with inferior infarction have demonstrable RV dysfunction, with hemodynamically significant RV failure in less than 10%.

Pathophysiology

Occlusion of the proximal right coronary artery interrupts flow in the branches to the free wall of the right ventricle and to distal branches to the inferior wall of the left ventricle. Ischemic injury or depression of the right ventricle causes a reduction in the transpulmonic flow of blood to the left ventricle. Inadequate LV filling pressure leads to a drop in cardiac output and to shock.

LV filling pressure may be in the normal range, but this may be misleading, and LV preload may actually be low. Abrupt dilatation of the ischemic right ventricle is limited by the rigid pericardium, and increased pressure in the pericardial space is transmitted to the LV. In fact, many have pulsus paradoxus, falsely suggesting tamponade. With animal models of RV infarction, hemodynamics improve when the pericardium is opened and pericardial crowding is relieved. Excessive fluid loading may increase pericardial pressure, further limiting diastolic return to the heart.

Many with RV infarction also have coexisting LV dysfunction and require an elevated LV filling pressure (above 15 to 18 mm Hg) to maintain stroke volume. LV dysfunction is severe enough in some patients that shock is the result of both RV and LV failure.

Clinical Presentation, Diagnosis, and Management

Consider RV infarction when there is hypotension complicating a large acute inferior MI (Table 5.10). On physical examination there are features of right heart failure, with jugular venous distention, and, with volume resuscitation, peripheral edema. As noted, there may be pulsus paradoxus (>10 mm Hg drop in systolic blood pressure with inspiration).

ST segment elevation in lead V_{4R} (a right precordial lead in the V_4 position) is sensitive and specific for RV ischemia. It indicates a worse prognosis with inferior MI, but right precordial ST elevation is not proof that shock is eminent; most with this finding do not develop shock. The echocardiogram shows dilatation of the right atrium and right ventricle and reduced contractility of the right ventricle, and it excludes pericardial effusion as the cause of pulsus paradoxus. Right heart catheterization documents elevation of the right atrial pressure, with minimal or no elevation of pulmonary artery pressure and low or normal LV filling pressure.

Treatment The RV infarction syndrome is prevented by early reperfusion. This is one more reason that large inferior MI is an indication for reperfusion therapy. Early right coronary artery reperfusion may hasten RV recovery, and even late reperfusion therapy with angioplasty has been recommended.

The initial treatment for hypotension during inferior MI is volume expansion. As long as there is no pulmonary congestion, a fluid challenge is safe, giving 200 mL normal saline per hour (or more) for a couple hours. If this does not correct hypotension, the patient needs hemodynamic monitoring with a pulmonary artery catheter. It is important to keep the pulmonary wedge pressure below 20 to 22 mm Hg to avoid pulmonary congestion. Above a certain level, the response of blood pressure and cardiac output flattens, indicating that increased pericardial pressure is limiting both RV and LV filling.

Intravenous nitroglycerin may aggravate hypotension because of reduced venous return to the heart. On the other hand, arterial vasodilator therapy may help, because lower left atrial and pulmonary artery pressures reduce RV afterload. When there is LV dysfunction in addition to RV dysfunction, treatment of hypotension with dobutamine is indicated. Improved contractility of the interventricular septum boosts RV stroke volume.

Refractory hypotension often improves with the IABP, particularly for those with coexisting LV dysfunction. In addition, balloon pumping improves coronary perfusion pressure, augmenting ventricular septal performance. Spontaneous recovery of RV function is common, and there is less chance of balloon dependence than there is with cardiogenic shock caused by LV injury.

Patients with RV infarction do poorly with bradycardia. For this reason, the threshold for treating bradyarrhythmias with AV sequential pacing is lower.

Clinical Course
Many with RV dysfunction have spontaneous improvement within 2 to 3 days. But it can be a more serious illness, and the mortality rate with RV infarction plus shock is 40%. Without shock it is less than 10%. Chronic right heart failure with peripheral edema and jugular venous distention is rare in survivors. This favorable long-term outlook is attributed to good collateral flow and the favorable oxygen supply–demand profile of the RV. Lower right heart pressure favors the transfer of coronary blood flow from the left ventricle to the right ventricle via collateral vessels.

Congestive Heart Failure
The risk of dying with heart diseases that affect adults is usually linked to LV systolic function, and low LVEF is the best predictor of mortality after MI. About 20% of the survivors of MI are disabled by heart failure within 6 years.

Pathophysiology
The cause of LV dysfunction after MI is loss of contractile units, translating to a loss of LVEF points. Occlusion of a large artery

supplying a broad myocardial region will have a greater influence on LVEF than occlusion of a small side branch.

Ischemia also increases myocardial stiffness, and diastolic dysfunction contributes to an increase in pulmonary wedge pressure and congestion.

Remodeling of the Left Ventricle (The Importance of LV Geometry) "Infarct expansion" and the associated change in LV geometry also contribute to heart failure. During the week after infarction, necrotic muscle softens and becomes mushy (for want of a better term). There is thinning of the LV wall with bulging and expansion of the soft infarct zone. This is most common with anterior MI, and the result is a change in the shape of the LV apex (Fig. 5.8). Instead of the normal elliptical shape, the LV apex has a rounded, mushroomlike shape. The most extreme form of this is LV aneurysm, where there is systolic bulging of the apex.

As subsequent healing takes place, scar is laid down in the "mold" provided by the altered infarct zone, resulting in a permanent alteration in shape. At that point the shape of the infarct zone is "cast in scar." The goal of afterload reduction therapy is prevention of early bulging, before scarring occurs.

Alteration in the shape of the apex has a negative effect on LV function. The radius of curvature of the left ventricle is increased. Because of the Laplace relationship (wall tension = pressure × radius), increased radius means an elevation of wall tension, and wall tension is the major determinant of myocardial oxygen demand. In addition, the bulging segment of myocardium "absorbs" some of the contractile energy of the left ventricle that would otherwise have gone toward ejection of blood.

Early reperfusion therapy preserves some muscle within the infarct zone and tends to prevent infarct expansion. When viewed in the operating room, the reperfused infarct zone has a marbled appearance, with patches of normal tissue mixed with injured muscle. This may explain an improvement in clinical course despite only minimal improvement in LVEF. Even with little preservation of contractile function, when enough muscle is saved to prevent infarct expansion, there is clinical benefit.

Treatment and Clinical Course

Effective (i.e., early) reperfusion therapy prevents heart failure. For those with large MI, including all patients with anterior MI,

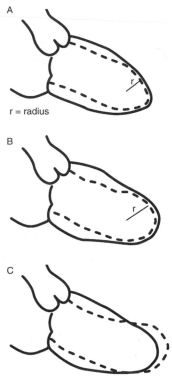

FIGURE 5.8. Three examples of left ventricular remodeling after MI (solid line, diastolic contour; dashed line, systolic contour). Patient A: The anterior wall is akinetic, but in diastole the left ventricle still has its ellipsoid shape (there has been no remodeling of LV shape). Patient B: In addition to anterior akinesis, the shape of the apex has changed so that it is rounded and more mushroomlike. This increases the radius (r) at the apex, and thus increases wall tension (see text). Patient C: There is an apical aneurysm. In addition to the rounded apex during diastole, there is aneurysmal bulging of the apex during systole. Not only is wall tension increased because of increased radius, but contractile energy is also "absorbed" by the bulging apex. This is the most extreme form of LV remodeling. (Reproduced by permission from Taylor GJ. Primary Care Management of Heart Disease. St. Louis, MO: Mosby, 2000.)

treatment with ACE inhibitors is the key to preventing infarct expansion, and treatment should be started within 24 hours of the onset of MI (Table 5.5). Trials testing ACE inhibition for smaller MIs have raised a possibility of short-term survival benefit, and some advocate their use for all patients with MI who do not have a contraindication (stay tuned for future studies). When there is LV dysfunction, defined as LVEF less than 40%, therapy should be continued long term, at least 3 years.

One in seven patients using ACE inhibitors stops the medicine because of cough. The angiotensin II blockers are good substitutes, having comparable effects when compared with captopril. Whether to recommend them as initial treatment will depend on the results of ongoing trials.

ACE inhibitor treatment tip: There is often concern about using ACE inhibitors or angiotensin II blockers in the patient with mild renal dysfunction, when the creatinine is above 1.5 mg/dL. Perhaps there is underlying renal artery stenosis, and therapy will aggravate it. What do you look for? First, blood pressure: A precipitous drop might indicate especially high plasma renin activity and underlying renal artery stenosis. Second, creatinine: Recheck it 24 to 48 hours after starting therapy. If the creatinine does not increase by more than 0.3 mg/dL, continue treatment. A small increase in creatinine necessitates repeat measurements. Be prepared to stop therapy if it continues to rise. A rise in creatinine with ACE inhibition is an indication to screen for renal artery stenosis.

Clinical Course Patients with heart failure during the course of acute infarction have a higher mortality risk (Table 5.2) and often develop chronic heart failure. They have complex ventricular arrhythmias (VAs), and sudden death is common. It is for this reason that careful monitoring of serum potassium and magnesium is critical for those requiring diuretics.

LV aneurysm is the most extreme case of infarct expansion. It is more common after anterior MI but may occur with inferior infarction. Persistent ST segment elevation may be an indicator of aneurysm, but it may also occur with large infarction in the absence of aneurysm. The diagnosis is easily made with an echocardiogram.

An aneurysm increases the mortality rate sixfold compared with those who have similar LVEF. Symptoms include the *clinical triad* of VAs, heart failure, and angina. Rupture of a mature aneurysm is uncommon. Surgical repair is a good option when it can be delayed for 4 to 6 weeks after MI (allowing development of tough enough scar tissue to hold sutures). The indication for aneurysmectomy is any one of the clinical triad plus a resectible aneurysm and a good opportunity for revascularization. Success depends on the contractility of the viable muscle, or the "residual EF" when the aneurysm is subtracted.

Arrhythmias
Complex VAs and Sudden Cardiac Death
It is important to distinguish between complex VAs that develop during the early hours of MI and those occurring in the late hospital phase (after days 3 to 4).

Early Ventricular Tachycardia (VT) or Ventricular Fibrillation (VF) VT or VF within the first day of MI appears to be an electrical phenomenon that is unrelated to infarct size. It may occur with small or large infarctions. Because the arrhythmia is not a marker of depressed LV function, it does not indicate poor long-term prognosis (providing, of course, that the patient survives the arrhythmia). This "electrical storm" usually resolves in a day.

Late Hospital-phase VT/VF The pathophysiology of complex VAs in the late hospital phase is different. They are limited to those with large MI. In fact, studies in the 1970s found that the best predictor of complex VAs was low LVEF, and the best predictor of low LVEF was complex VAs on a predischarge 24-hour monitor. After MI, documenting normal LV function indicates a low risk of complex VAs, and it is unnecessary to get a 24-hour monitor as a screen for ventricular ectopy.

Patients with a depressed left ventricle and complex VAs tend to have them all the time. They are not sporadic as is commonly the case with supraventricular tachycardia. A single 24-hour monitor done at random is enough to document complex VAs (frequent VPBs, pairs or nonsustained VT). A normal 24-hour monitor excludes them with fair certainty. There is no need to repeat monitoring for fear of having missed VAs.

Treatment
Lidocaine lowers the risk of VF, but as noted, it is no longer recommended as prophylactic therapy during acute MI. It should be given when there are frequent ventricular ectopic beats during the first day after MI. When lidocaine fails to prevent recurrence of VT or VF, intravenous amiodarone, bretyllium, or procainamide may be effective. An occasional patient with refractory VT will respond to intravenous magnesium.

TABLE 5.11. **Lessons from the Cardiac Arrhythmia Suppression Trial (CAST)**

1. CAST demonstrated that proarrhythmia is more important than expected. Suppression of asymptomatic PVCs or nonsustained ventricular tachycardia (NSVT) after MI with class IC drugs increased the risk of sudden death.
2. CAST did not study class IA drugs (quinidine or procainamide). They also have proarrhythmic effects, and the safety of long-term therapy is uncertain.
3. Suppression of PVCs on an ambulatory monitor did not predict improved survival with drug therapy. The mechanisms responsible for PVCs may differ from those causing sustained arrhythmias and sudden death.
4. The rate, length, and frequency of nonsustained VT had no influence on prognosis. A single 3-beat burst of VT at a rate of 120/min carried the same prognostic weight as multiple 8 to 10 beat runs at 150/min.
5. An exception to the above, VT rates <100 beats/min indicated a mortality rate lower than VT rates above 100/min.
6. CAST did *not* include patients with normal LV function. With normal LVEF after MI, treatment of asymptomatic PVCs and NSVT with drugs other than beta-blockers is not indicated.
7. CAST did not study patients without CAD. The data may not apply to others with LV dysfunction (e.g., dilated cardiomyopathy).
8. CAST did not exclude possible efficacy of other drugs such as amiodarone.

Late Hospital-phase and Postdischarge VA Those with sustained VT, VT causing syncope, or VF should have electrophysiologic evaluation (see Chapter 6). There has been controversy about prophylactic antiarrhythmic therapy for the patient with low LVEF and complex VAs. This group has the highest mortality in the year after MI, and more than half of the deaths are sudden. The first step in treatment is to exclude conditions that may aggravate ventricular ectopy, including recurrent ischemia and electrolyte abnormalities. Look for low magnesium and potassium.

The Cardiac Arrhythmia Suppression Trial specifically studied the role of antiarrhythmic drug therapy after MI for patients with depressed LVEF and complex ectopy, and it substantially changed our approach to therapy (Table 5.11). A pilot study screened a number of drugs and indentified those best at suppressing VAs on 24-hour monitors. Encainide, flecainide, and moricizine were the winners, whereas quinidine and procainamide were less effective. The next and largest phase of the study compared the most effective drugs with placebo. The result was surprising: Death or cardiac arrest was 2.64 times higher with drug treatment than with placebo. The proarrhythmic effects of these drugs were more important than expected. Membrane active agents suppress ectopy on the monitor, but they do not prevent sudden death.

Interestingly, *beta-blockers* have the opposite effect. As a rule, they do not suppress ectopy on the 24-hour monitor, but the incidence of sudden death is lower. Apparently there is a difference between suppressing VPBs and preventing sustained VAs, including VF. For asymptomatic ventricular ectopy, beta blockade is the treatment of choice.

You may consider amiodarone for the patient with VT who, for whatever reason, is not a candidate for an implantable defibrillator. Canadian and European trials showed no reduction cardiac death, but both found a reduction in arrhythmic death. In the Canadian trial, reduction in arrhythmic death was greatest among patients with congestive heart failure and those with a history of multiple MIs (as usual, those with the highest risk had the greatest benefit).

At one time arrhythmia specialists were using electrophysiology study to select the best antiarrhythmic agent; VT was induced in the electrophysiology lab, and different drugs were tested until one was found that blocked induced VT, so-called guided therapy. The largest randomized trial of this approach found no benefit with guided drug therapy. In the same study, implantable defibrillator therapy substantially reduced the risk of cardiac arrest and death.

So where do we stand at this point? First, patients with long runs of VT or symptomatic VT should have electrophysiologic testing. Implantable defibrillator therapy is life saving for those with inducible sustained VT. Second, others with brief spells of nonsustained VT and those who do not have inducible VT in the electrophysiology laboratory should be treated with beta-blockers. Finally, amiodarone can be justified for those with heart failure and nonsustained VT when other therapies are not feasible.

Amiodarone is the only membrane active agent that does not appear to *increase* the risk of sudden death in patients with previous MI and depressed LV function. There are a few clinical settings where it is commonly used. First, it may prevent symptomatic VT, and control of symptoms is one indication. Second, those with an implantable defibrillator need to have VT suppressed to prevent frequent firing of the device. Finally, amiodarone is effective for treatment and prevention of atrial fibrillation; it can be used for this purpose in the post-MI patient with depressed LV function with less risk of sudden death than other drugs.

Atrial Tachyarrhythmias

Atrial fibrillation, supraventricular tachycardia, and sinus tachycardia tend to develop in patients with large MI. They are markers of low LVEF, and thus identify poor prognosis. Recognition and treatment are reviewed in Chapter 6.

Bradyarrhythmias

The prognosis with heart block is determined by the location of block. As a rule, when conduction is blocked at the level of the AV node, the take-over pacemaker is reliable and has an intrinsic rate above 40 beats/min. The AV node usually recovers, and permanent pacing is seldom needed. Infranodal block is a much bigger problem, with a slow take-over pacer and little chance of recovery. It is an indication for a permanent pacemaker. *In general, a narrow QRS complex indicates nodal block and a wide QRS means infranodal block.*

Inferior MI commonly causes heart block. The right coronary artery supplies the AV node, and heart block is thus nodal, with a narrow QRS complex. Recovery is the rule, and pacing is seldom needed.

When *anterior MI* causes heart block, the mechanism is injury to nerves running through the interventricular septum. Block is infranodal, the QRS complex is wide with a bundle branch block pattern, and the prognosis for recovery is poor. A permanent pacemaker is needed. This is not a common issue, because patients with anterior MI and heart block have huge MIs and usually die from cardiogenic shock before a pacemaker is needed.

Recurrent Myocardial Ischemia

The incidence of postinfarction angina is 20% to 30%. It is more common in patients with non-Q wave MI, because the infarct is incomplete and the infarct artery is tightly stenosed and unstable. Coronary occlusion and recurrent MI are common. Other risk factors for recurrent ischemia are obesity, female sex, diabetes, and early peaking CK (an indicator of spontaneous thrombolysis).

Patients with MI and ST elevation treated with thrombolytic therapy also have "incomplete infarction" and are at risk for angina or recurrence ("completion") of the MI. Primary angioplasty leaves the patient with a more stable artery, and there is less chance of reocclusion and reinfarction than there is after thrombolytic therapy. But the risk of recurrent ischemia is still appreciable, and careful monitoring is needed during the 2 to 3 days after the procedure.

Reocclusion of the infarct artery and "extension" of the infarct has a bad effect on prognosis. Mortality and heart failure are both increased. This holds true with clinically silent infarct artery reocclusion.

Remember that silent reocclusion of the infarct artery is common. In fact, it is probably more common than symptomatic reocclusion, because nociceptive dysfunction is the rule following transient coronary artery occlusion. Consider recurrent ischemia if a patient has an unexplained increase in ventricular ectopy, has more elevation of ST segments on the telemetry ECG, or has unexpected or vague symptoms such as anxiety, restlessness, or dyspnea. Reocclusion of the infarct artery is promptly identified by reelevation of the ST segments on a 12-lead ECG.

Management
Aspirin and beta-blockers both lower the risk of recurrent angina and infarction. Diltiazem has that effect on patients with non-Q MI. Nitrates have not been shown to prevent ischemia after MI. After reperfusion therapy, most infarct artery reocclusion is missed. Prevention of this complication is the rationale for angiography and revascularization, which are aimed at "pacifying" the unstable vessel.

If there is recurrence of angina at rest, get an ECG during pain to document new ST segment changes. Standard medical therapy may be applied—even before the ECG—including sublingual nitroglycerin, beta-blockers (intravenous or oral), aspirin, and heparin. Unless there is a dramatic response to nitroglycerin, urgent angiography and angioplasty are the best treatments for recurrence of ischemia. Thrombolytic therapy may be used for reocclusion, but we consider it a second choice because of the higher risk of myocardial rupture with late thrombolysis.

Pericarditis
Fibrinous Pericarditis Early Post-MI
Transient pericarditis is common during the first week of transmural infarction (usually within 3 days). It is more common with

large MI, occurring in 25% of those with Q wave infarction and less than 10% with non-Q MI. Limiting infarct size with early reperfusion therapy may prevent it.

Most patients have a transient friction rub without pain. A few have inflammation severe enough to cause pain that raises the possibility of postinfarction angina. The history and physical examination make the diagnosis straightforward in most cases. The pain is typical of pericardits and different from the pain of the recent MI. It is "pleuritic" and improves with sitting and leaning forward. Radiation of the pain to the trapezius ridge suggests pericarditis. Unlike viral pericarditis, the ECG is usually unchanged, without diffuse ST segment elevation. Pneumonitis is uncommon, as inflammation is limited to the pericardium.

The echocardiogram may show a small pericardial effusion. Tamponade is rare; when it occurs, it is usually due to ventricular rupture or to hemopericardium. Because antiplatelet and anticoagulant therapy are commonly used after MI, there is concern about transforming fibrinous pericarditis to hemopericardium and tamponade. This is an unusual complication, and mild pericarditis is not considered an indication for stopping anticoagulants when the patient is already on them. Furthermore, I would not hesitate to start anticoagulant therapy when the need is great. For example, recent angioplasty or stent placement, discovery of an LV thrombus, or development of unstable angina would weigh in favor of anticoagulation, despite the presence of a friction rub.

The best treatment for early pericarditis is aspirin at doses that suppress inflammation (650 mg at 4- to 6-hour intervals). Both steroids and nonsteroidal anti-inflammatory drugs may increase the risk of rupture when given early after MI. They may promote infarct expansion as well.

Pericarditis is usually transient, has no direct clinical consequences, and does not recur. If a rub and fever redevelop more than 10 days after MI, it is Dressler's syndrome, a different illness. On the other hand, early pericarditis is a marker of larger infarction and thus a more complicated clinical course.

Late Pericarditis: Dressler's Syndrome

This post-MI syndrome is fibrinous pericarditis that is localized to the region of infarction. It is much less common than when it was first described in 1957, now occurring in about 1% of patients with MI. Symptoms begin 10 days to 8 weeks after MI. In addition to typical pericarditis, there is evidence of generalized inflammation with fever, malaise, aching muscles (a flulike syndrome), elevation of the sedimentation rate, leukocytosis, and pericardial effusion. Pneumonitis is possible, with patchy infiltrates on the chest x-ray. It is a rare cause of pericardial tamponade. Clinically, it is similar to the postpericardiotomy syndrome that occurs after heart surgery, an illness that you are more likely to encounter in a general medical practice.

There is no single test that confirms the diagnosis. You are safe making the call based on the clinical picture and sedimentation rate above 80 to 100 mm/hr. A normal sedimentation rate makes Dressler's syndrome unlikely.

The best treatment is high-dose aspirin when pericarditis occurs within 4 weeks of MI. An occasional patient with severe inflammation requires steroids, but we try to avoid them because of possible effects on scar formation. Treatment with steroids or nonsteroidal anti-inflammatory agents within 2 weeks of MI increases the risk of rupture. The risk 2 to 4 weeks after MI is uncertain. After 4 weeks, steroids and nonsteroidal anti-inflammatory agents are considered safe.

With anti-inflammatory therapy, there is resolution of symptoms within a week. I stop therapy a week later or when inflammation has resolved. A falling sedimentation rate would favor stopping therapy. Continued treatment will not prevent recurrence. Some patients have recurrent symptoms, and treatment can be restarted. Later episodes are not as severe or as close together as earlier spells. In time the illness seems to burn itself out, and it is uncommon for flare-ups to develop more than 6 months after MI. (This describes the natural history of the postpericardiotomy syndrome as well.)

LV Thrombus and Peripheral Embolization

Without anticoagulation, mural thrombus develops in as many as 20% with Q wave MI, and the incidence rises to 40% with anterior MI. It is more common with large infarction. About 10% of those with LV thrombus have peripheral embolization. Thus, the risk of embolization ranges from 1% to 4% with acute MI, depending on the size and location of infarction.

The pathogenesis of ventricular clot is uncertain. A loss of wall motion may lead to stagnation of blood in contact with the surface; normal contraction keeps blood moving along (that seems the case when comparing atrial fibrillation with flutter). It has also been suggested that inflammation of the endocardial surface of infarcted muscle may be thrombogenic. Embolization is more likely when a clot is mobile, protrudes more into the chamber, or is large enough (to be seen in multiple echo views).

Management

Heparin during acute MI lowers the chance of LV thrombus by 50%. There have been no trials large enough to show a reduction of peripheral embolization. Thrombolytic therapy also reduces the chance of thrombus formation, but there has been a report of late thrombolytic therapy dislodging an LV thrombus, shaking an embolus loose.

The transthoracic echocardiogram is sensitive and specific for the diagnosis of LV thrombus; it is not necessary to do a transesophageal study. The current recommendations for prevention and therapy are outlined in Table 5.7.

Pulmonary Embolus

The best prevention for venous thrombus and pulmonary embolism is early ambulation. When MI was treated with prolonged bedrest, pulmonary embolus was responsible for 10% of deaths; it is a rare cause of death after MI presently. Patients at high risk should have prophylaxis with subcutaneous heparin (Table 5.7). The Practice Guidelines call for routine treatment of all patients during the first 2 days in hospital (for the unusual patient not receiving full-dose heparin).

New Murmur after MI (Table 5.10)
Rupture of the Interventricular Septum
(Acute Ventricular Septal Defect)

Acute mitral regurgitation and ventricular septal defect (VSD) are the causes of new systolic murmur after MI. The incidence of septal rupture with MI is about 2%. It is more common with advanced age, hypertension, and poorly developed collateral circulation; most have multivessel CAD. Like free wall rupture, thrombolytic therapy more than 12 hours from the onset of MI may predispose to rupture of the septum.

The interventricular septum is supplied by branches from both the anterior descending and posterior descending arteries, the two coronary branches that encircle the septum in the inter-ventricular groove. Thus, either anterior or inferior MI may cause septal rupture. The prognosis is worse with inferior infarction, possibly because the basal location of the defect makes surgical repair more difficult. A VSD caused by anterior MI is positioned nearer the LV apex. Proximal septal rupture is rare, probably because ischemic injury that extensive causes cardiogenic shock and death before rupture occurs.

VSD develops during the first day of MI in 20%, and most occur within the first week. A loud, harsh, holosystolic murmur is the rule, and many have a thrill. Biventricular failure follows. With medical therapy, half die within a week, and 85% by 2 weeks.

Management A new murmur is an indication for an urgent echocardiogram. The Doppler study demonstrates flow across the ventricular septum and excludes mitral regurgitation. *The next step is prompt transfer for angiography and surgical repair.*

While transfer is being arranged, blood pressure may be sup-ported with catecholamines and congestion treated with diuret-ics. Hypotension or a low cardiac output syndrome would be indications for the IABP. Right heart catheterization confirms the diagnosis: The oxygen saturation in the pulmonary artery is higher than in the vena cava and right atrium (there is a "step-up" in oxygen saturation at the level of the right ventricle).

Immediate surgical repair is indicated for the usual patient with VSD who is dependent on catecholamine and/or IABP sup-port. Surgical success is predicted by good ventricular function and brief duration of shock. A rare patient stabilizes without developing shock. In such cases, surgery may be delayed 3 to 4 weeks, hoping that partially healed tissue will be easier to repair. During this time careful monitoring is needed, because rapid deterioration is possible.

Acute Mitral Regurgitation

The incidence of papillary muscle rupture with MI is 1%. The posteromedial papillary muscle is supplied by the right coronary artery, and the anterolateral muscle by the circumflex branch.

Inferior MI is a more common cause of mitral regurgitation than lateral infarction. Unlike VSD, a tiny MI may cause mitral regurgitation, because infarction of just the tip of a papillary muscle may lead to rupture. The patient may have single-vessel CAD.

The onset of heart failure and pulmonary congestion is abrupt. Many have a loud holosystolic murmur but no thrill (a thrill suggests VSD). When cardiac output and blood pressure are low, the murmur may be soft. Unlike chronic mitral regurgitation, there is no S_3 gallop. In fact, there may be an S_4 gallop, because the ventricle has not dilated.

When a patient with a small MI unexpectedly develops heart failure, get an echocardiogram to rule out mitral regurgitation, regardless of the presence or absence of a murmur.

The echocardiogram demonstrates mitral regurgitation and often a flail mitral leaflet. LV function may be near normal. The pulmonary wedge pressure tracing typically shows a tall V wave, analogous to the V wave in the venous pulse in patients with tricuspid regurgitation.

When pulmonary congestion is severe and there is low cardiac output, nitroprusside and the IABP provide a bridge to surgery. Immediate surgical repair is indicated. The biggest problem is the failure to recognize mitral regurgitation as the cause of heart failure.

Rupture of the Ventricular Free Wall

Rupture of the free wall of the left ventricle is the second most common cause of death in patients hospitalized with MI (after LV failure) and is responsible for 10% of deaths. It occurs 3 to 7 days after MI, at about the same time as acute VSD or mitral regurgitation. At this time after MI, the necrotic infarct zone is softest. It commonly happens after a first MI and may occur with small or large infarctions (usually anterior or lateral in location). Single-vessel CAD and poorly developed collaterals are common. Risk factors for rupture are late coronary thrombolysis (more than 12 hours from the onset of MI), hypertension, and advanced age. But it is not uncommon in young patients. Steroids and nonsteroidal anti-inflammatory agents probably increase the risk of rupture, but this is uncertain. Because anti-inflammatory therapy alters healing and scar formation, it probably should be avoided for a month after MI.

The clinical picture is one of acute tamponade and death. I have observed a number of cases with the patient in hospital. There may be mild agitation or other vague symptoms just before rupture, but no anginal chest pain. Telemetry shows no arrhythmia. After the patient collapses, there is electromechanical dissociation (also called pulseless electrical activity). Resuscitation is unsuccessful. There is not enough time for emergency surgery. This is a cause of sudden cardiac death for which there is no successful treatment. There are case reports describing emergency surgical repair and survival, but I have never seen it, even when we made the clinical diagnosis.

Note that rupture may occur soon after discharge from the hospital and often in a patient with small MI. For this reason, I tell patients with small infarction that the prognosis is good (especially when LV function is normal) but also indicate that there are rare complications of MI during the first month that prevent my guaranteeing a benign course.

Pseudoaneurysm An occasional patient with rupture has it contained by adherent pericardium, probably because of inflammation of the infarcted muscle and overlying pericardium. There is usually clot within the bulging aneurysmal sack that provides support but that also may embolize. A pseuoaneurysm tends to have a narrow neck where it communicates with the left ventricle, distinguishing it from a true aneurysm. It may become quite large and may rupture. There are no clinical findings that indicate its presence, and it is usually an unexpected finding on an echocardiogram. Because of possible rupture, surgical repair is indicated.

When you hear of the rare case of free wall rupture that was successfully treated, it probably involved rupture with some degree of containment by the pericardium, preventing tamponade, circulatory collapse, and immediate death.

LONG-TERM TREATMENT AFTER MI _____

Risk Stratification
Patients who are preparing to leave the hospital after MI face the possibility of sudden cardiac death, recurrent infarction, heart failure, or peripheral embolization during the next year (Table 5.12). The current standard of care includes laboratory studies to identify those at high risk for these late complications of MI plus

TABLE 5.12. Potential Complications During the Year After MI

Complication	Screening Study	Prophylaxis
Sudden cardiac death (VF)	Echo or RNA to measure LVEF; 24-hour ambulatory monitor predischarge for those with depressed LVEF. EPS for those with sustained VT.	Beta blockade, aspirin to prevent ischemia, normalize electrolytes, revascularization if there is active ischemia, AICD if sustained VT is induced during EPS.
Recurrent ischemia or MI	Stress ECG with or without imaging study for low-risk patients (see text), angiography for those at high risk.	Aspirin and beta blockade for all patients; revascularization for those with active ischemia.
Heart failure, progression of LV dysfunction (remodeling)	Echocardiogram for those with anterior MI or evidence for large MI.	ACE inhibitor therapy.
LV thrombus and peripheral embolization	Echocardiogram for those with anterior MI or large MI.	Warfarin when thrombus is documented; antiplatelet therapy is less effective.
Progression of CAD	Lipid analysis (see text for timing)	The goal of therapy is LDL < 100 mg/dL; reductase inhibitor therapy is usually needed.
Cardiac rupture	No screening possible.	None known.

EPS, electrophysiologic study; LDL, low-density lipoprotein; RNA, radionuclide angiogram.

TABLE 5.13. Noninvasive Screening Studies for Complex VAs after MI

Study	Comment
Measurement of LVEF (echocardiogram, radionuclide angiogram, cardiac cath)	Those with poor LV function are at risk for complex ventricular ectopy and sudden death. It would be unusual to find serious VAs in one with normal LVEF.
24-hour ambulatory monitor (Holter monitor)	Monitoring is not necessary for those with small infarction and normal LVEF. Patients at high risk for sudden death tend to have complex VAs throughout each day. A single 24-hour monitor is an adequate screen.
Signal-averaged ECG (SAECG)*	Computer summation of a large number of QRS complexes allows measurement of the low-voltage "late-potential" at the tail-end of the QRS in patients with reentrant VAs. This current may come from the reentrant circuit. Late-potentials correlate with low LVEF and complex VAs after MI.
Heart rate variability (HRV)*	Large MI and low LVEF leads to decreased parasympathetic (vagal) tone. Vagal discharge is responsible for sinus arrhythmia, the normal respiratory variation in heart rate (or HRV). With loss of vagal tone, HRV decreases (the rhythm, and the RR interval, become more regular). *Technique:* A large number of RR intervals are collected by a computer on the ECG machine and averaged. The *standard deviation* of the mean RR interval is a measure of variation, or HRV: Low HRV correlates with low LVEF and complex VAs.

*Based on available studies, it does not appear that HRV or the SAECG add novel information about prognosis over and above that provided by LVEF and Holter monitoring. They have been suggested as alternative screening techniques. RR interval, the distance (or time) between two R waves on the ECG.

treatment to prevent them. Think of Table 5.12 as a "menu" that you can review at the time of hospital discharge; it is a broad review of the Practice Guidelines from the American Heart Association.

Sudden Cardiac Death After MI

A normal LVEF (above 50% to 55% on an echocardiogram) almost excludes the possibility of sudden arrhythmic death. For this reason, measurement of LVEF is a key step in screening for possible sudden cardiac death (Tables 5.12 and 5.13). If the LVEF is low, get a 24-hour ambulatory monitor.

A practical question is whether telemetry on the ward just before discharge may be substituted for tape recorder monitoring. If the telemetry system does not have memory that allows review of 24 hours of monitoring or if monitoring depends on a nurse watching the screen, then it is not adequate. Newer telemetry systems with expanded memory and review capabilities are reasonable substitutes for tape recorder monitoring, if they are used properly.

Newer screening techniques for arrhythmia potential include the signal-averaged ECG and measures of heart rate variability (Table 5.13). Abnormal studies correlate with low LVEF and an increased risk of complex VAs. Although relatively inexpensive and easy to perform, they are not widely available, and their role in the screening process is not yet established.

The management of VAs after MI has been discussed. A couple points are worth reemphasizing: Beta blockade lowers the risk of sudden death and is indicated for all patients after MI, particularly those with nonsustained VT. Patients with depressed LV function often are on diuretics. Meticulous attention to serum potassium and magnesium (the overlooked electrolyte) are critical elements of arrhythmia prevention.

Residual or Recurrent Myocardial Ischemia

All patients with MI should be screened for the possibility of a future ischemic event, regardless of how small or uncomplicated the MI. A meta-analyis found that ST segment depression on a stress ECG was 44% sensitive in predicting cardiac death or reinfarction within the year after MI. Sensitivity improved to 80% with an exercise perfusion scan, to 71% with a pharmacologic perfusion scan, to 62% with an exercise echocardiogram, and to 55% with a pharmacologic stress echo (see Chapter 4 for a description of these tests). Most studies of exercise testing after MI excluded patients with poor LV function. A large MI, particularly if complicated by heart failure, is a relative contraindication to early exercise testing, and angiography is safer. Angiography also is also preferable for those with angina after MI.

Can the low-risk patient have an exercise ECG alone, or must you add an imaging study? The practice guidelines do not indicate a preference, despite recognition that imaging studies add sensitivity. I do not believe that you could be faulted for doing a symptom-limited exercise ECG in a setting of small uncomplicated first MI and doing no further workup if the study is negative and exercise tolerance is good (more than 7 minutes on the treadmill using the Bruce protocol).

A Warning About Imaging Studies

You should be aware that these techniques are operator dependent. The studies demonstrating their accuracy were performed
in centers that have dedicated teams doing nuclear cardiology or
echocardiography full time. Although not widely discussed, there
is a problem when translating these results to some practice settings, where scans may be read by a radiologist with little training
or experience with nuclear cardiac imaging. Local experience
often dictates the choice of study. If you have an experienced echo
team, use echo. If there is more experience with nuclear studies,
that is the choice. If your hospital has little or no experience with
either, be aware that buying a nuclear camera does not mean that
you will automatically get dependable results.

Timing of the Exercise Study

It is a fielder's choice. Testing while the patient is in hospital,
within 4 to 6 days of MI, rules out ischemia that may occur early
after discharge. There is also the logistic advantage of getting
everything done while the patient is still in the hospital. But the
early exercise test should not push the patient hard (the target
heart rate is usually 120 beats/min). Exercise tolerance is not
tested with early study.

The advantage of later testing, more than 10 days after MI,
is that exercise tolerance may be measured with a symptom-limited test. That is important, because poor exercise tolerance indicates poor prognosis and is even more sensitive than ST segment
depression on the stress ECG. For the low-risk patient with a
small, apparently completed MI, you may want the more complete study done 10 to 14 days after MI. If there is uncertainty about
the patient's stability, a predischarge study would be preferred.

Incomplete MI and Indications for Angiography

Patients with non-Q wave infarction and patients with Q-wave
MI treated with thrombolytic therapy usually have unstable coronary plaque. There is viable muscle in the region supplied by the
diseased artery, and the infarct is considered "incomplete." They
are at high risk for occlusion of the infarct vessel and probably
should have angiography. Delaying transfer for angiography
makes no sense; there is a chance that occlusion and reinfarction
will occur while the patient languishes (usually in the middle of

the night). The day after acute MI is a good time for transfer, when early VAs and chest pain have resolved. Early transfer also positions the patient in the catheterization lab queue, ensuring timely study.

Therapy to Prevent Recurrent Ischemia or Infarction

Those with high-risk coronary anatomy usually have revascularization. Others are treated with aspirin and beta-blockers. There are two situations where *not* prescribing beta blockade after MI may be reasonable: 1) single-vessel CAD, a small and completed MI, where the risk of future ischemia and arrhythmia is low, and 2) after revascularization, where the risk of future ischemia is low.

Progression of Atherosclerosis

Long-term prognosis for the low-risk patient is determined by progression of disease. The best way to prevent this and to improve survival is to push the low-density-lipoprotein cholesterol below 100 mg/dL. That goal has become the standard of care for all with documented CAD. Reaching it usually requires therapy with reductase inhibitors or niacin. (Note that 100 mg/dL may not be low enough. Ongoing trials should identify the optimal LDL level.)

What You Cannot Screen for

Other late complications of MI have been discussed. Do not forget that after completing the evaluation process and identifying the low-risk patient, there is still a small risk of myocardial rupture as a cause of sudden death. Although it is right to emphasize an optimistic prognosis, you cannot and therefore should not guarantee it.

Exercise Therapy and Activity After MI
Training Effects

The best measure of cardiovascular fitness is VO_2max, or the maximum amount of oxygen the body is able to use during exercise. This can be measured during a metabolic exercise test with a device that collects expired air and measures oxygen uptake (as well as minute ventilation and carbon dioxide production). VO_2max is influenced by the oxygen-carrying capacity of blood (which declines with anemia), pulmonary function, and an ability to

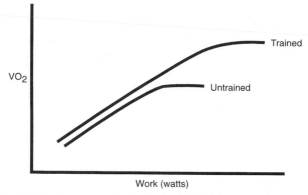

FIGURE 5.9. Oxygen uptake by the body (VO_2) increases during work. Everyone's cardiopulmonary reserve has a limit, and VO_2 reaches a plateau. This is VO_2max, which defines the level of fitness; the trained individual has a much higher VO_2max. Heart rate, blood pressure, and minute ventilation also increase with work. However, at any level of work (or level of VO_2), they are lower for the trained person. Thus, the trained person has a more efficient body and higher cardiopulmonary reserve. (Reproduced by permission from Taylor GJ. Primary Care Management of Heart Disease. St. Louis, MO, Mosby: 2000.)

raise cardiac output. Notice that the curve flattens when VO_2max is reached (Fig. 5.9). At this VO_2 plateau, continued exercise is accomplished with a disproportionate rise in minute ventilation and CO_2 production relative to oxygen uptake (VO_2). In fact, this "anaerobic threshold" is reached some time before the VO_2 plateau and is identified as the point where CO_2 production increases (usually at about 40% to 70% of VO_2max).

Trained distance athletes have a high VO_2max, partly the result of greater cardiac reserve. (World class athletes are genetically gifted with VO_2max above 70 mL/kg/min.) Measurable differences with training include increased blood volume, LV dilatation, and therefore increased stroke volume. With training, skeletal muscles become more efficient, with an increased capacity for oxidative metabolism. For any given level of VO_2 (oxygen utilization by the body, in mL/kg/min), the trained individual is doing a similar amount of external work. However, that level of work (and VO_2) is accomplished with lower heart rate, blood pressure, and minute ventilation. That is a rough description of the "training effect."

On the other hand, exercise training has little measurable effect on myocardial contractility. Small improvements in LVEF have been demonstrated with high intensity exercise, but not at levels of exercise commonly used in cardiac rehabilitation programs.

The training effect is achieved by patients with heart disease in aerobic exercise programs. VO_2 max is higher, and for a given work load or VO_2, heart rate is lower. For a patient with severe exercise limitations, a small improvement in VO_2max may be the difference between total disability and a return to simple activities outside the home.

Other benefits of exercise include weight loss, better control of diabetes, and increased high-density lipoprotein cholesterol. The psychological benefits cannot be overemphasized. Patients in formal exercise programs recover more quickly and are able to resume normal physical activity sooner.

Effects of Exercise Therapy on Survival Multiple studies have attempted to show a survival benefit of cardiac rehabilitation. Generally, they have not yielded statistical proof that exercise therapy reduces mortality. These are tough studies to do. There is a lot of crossover of control patients into exercise programs, and the studies have been small with short-term follow-up. The magnitude of survival benefit in these studies has been similar to that found in beta-blocker trials, but with too few patients to achieve statistical significance.

Patient Selection for Exercise Therapy An important change in recent years is the discovery that patients with cardiac dysfunction benefit from exercise training. In fact, those with lower VO_2max tend to have a greater benefit in terms of percentage increase in exercise tolerance. We commonly send patients with low LVEF and mildly symptomatic heart failure to cardiac rehabilitation. In such cases the exercise prescription and surveillance during training are critical.

A baseline exercise test is the basis for an exercise prescription. The major *contraindications* to training are exercise-induced ischemia, arrhythmias, and heart failure. When these complications of exercise are identified on the baseline treadmill study, exercise training is avoided until they are corrected. Correction may not be possible. Those with persistent ischemia despite optimal therapy may proceed with exercise therapy but at levels well below the ischemic threshold (see Chapter 4). Similarly, a patient with heart failure may do well with shorter periods of exercise and a lower target heart rate.

Patients with the combination of *heart failure plus ischemia* have the highest risk of complications during exercise training. At the low level of exercise they tolerate, they seldom achieve a conditioning effect.

The Exercise Prescription A baseline treadmill test is needed to design a training program. It allows screening for exercise-induced ischemia or arrhythmias and definition of maximum heart rate and exercise tolerance. The symptom-limited exercise study done a couple weeks after MI provides all the required data.

Conditioning is dependent on the frequency, intensity, and length of exercise sessions, and those are the elements of the "exercise prescription." The minimum *frequency* for cardiac fitness is three sessions per week. Once the patient is in shape, the target *intensity* is exercise to 85% of the maximum heart rate (based on the treadmill study). At the beginning the target rate should be lower, about 65% of the maximum rate, and this can be slowly advanced during the first 6 weeks of exercise. Less perceived exertion with a given exercise indicates that the intensity of exercise can be increased. The ideal *length* of exercise is 40 minutes of aerobic conditioning, preceded by a 10-minute warm-up and followed by a 10-minute cool-down.

The type of exercise is tailored to the patient. It should be aerobic. Strength training, and especially isometric exercise, is avoided because it causes a disproportionate rise in blood pressure when compared with the increase in heart rate. Most are comfortable with dynamic leg training (walking or bicycling).

Supervised group exercise offers a number of benefits. An inexperienced patient learns how to exercise and often learns a bit about exercise physiology. Risk factors are addressed in the group setting. Unanticipated difficulties with exercise are detected. Many programs intermittently monitor even low-risk patients, screening for exercise-induced arrhythmias. Exercise groups tend to bond, and the community provides psychosocial support, as does the rehabilitation staff. Most insurance benefit programs provide 8 to 12 weeks of formal cardiac rehabilitation after MI.

Many patients exercise at home, outside the supervised setting. This is safe for those who do not have exercise-induced ischemia or arrhythmias. They should exercise to a prescribed target heart rate. It helps to suggest limits on perceived exertion as well. I tell patients that as long as they can talk, whistle, or sing, they probably are not pushing too hard.

Safety of Exercise Training Aerobic exercise, as prescribed above, is safe for those without severe LV dysfunction or exercise-induced ischemia or arrhythmia.

High-risk patients are safest exercising in a supervised group with ECG monitoring. High risk is identified by symptoms or objective signs of any of the following: severe LV dysfunction, heart failure, exercise-induced ischemia, complex VAs, poor exercise tolerance, hypotension with exercise, or inability to self-monitor heart rate. Such patients may benefit from participation in a supervised group program for longer than the usual 8 to 12 weeks.

Supervised group exercise with either continuous or intermittent monitoring has a good safety record. The risk of death is 1.3 per million patient hours of exercise, and of resuscitated cardiac arrest, 8.9 per million patient hours.

Counseling the Patient About Common Physical Activity

The exercise test done within 3 weeks of MI provides reassurance for you and your patient about the safety of exercise. The absence of exercise-induced ischemia and/or arrhythmias indicates that normal activities of daily living and a regular exercise program may be started with safety.

Heart Rate 120 beats/min It is a number worth remembering. Ambulatory monitoring studies early after uncomplicated MI have shown that activities such as walking up stairs and light housework push the heart rate to about 120 beats/min, but rarely higher. That is one reason that predischarge exercise testing is performed with a target heart rate of 120 beats/min. Tell the patient that it is a "safety test." Reaching 120 beats/min with no ECG abnormality or symptoms indicates that walking up stairs, carrying a bag of groceries, sweeping the kitchen floor, or making a bed will also be safe.

Sexual Activity The same monitoring studies found that sex with one's usual partner and in a familiar setting pushes the heart rate to 120 beats/min. On the other hand, sex in a novel setting or with an unfamiliar partner produces a much higher heart rate response. If the patient can walk up stairs without symptoms, sexual intercourse is safe. Checking the pulse rate after sex provides useful objective information.

Patients who are being treated medically for angina after MI may find that sublingual nitroglycerin just before sex prevents symptoms. There is no reason to recommend this for those who do not have angina.

Viagra A number of middle-aged men will have used fildenafil (Viagra) before MI. The drug blocks degradation of nitric oxide and thus has vasodilating properties. It is not contraindicated in patients with CAD or after MI. On the other hand, it is contraindicated for those taking nitrates, because it enhances the hypotensive effects of nitroglycerin and may cause syncope. This may be a concern for the patient with angina who is not taking long-acting nitrates but who uses intermittent sublingual nitroglycerin. If sexual activity provokes angina, nitroglycerin could be dangerous after taking Viagra.

Follow-up After MI and Expected Clinical Course

Most patients experience easy fatigue and a general loss of energy after MI. Those who have had moderate to large MI and who have depressed LV function are fatigued because of limits on cardiac performance. But patients with small infarction and normal LVEF also experience a loss of vigor. Tell them that this is the usual state during early healing after MI and that energy levels will return to normal a couple months after the infarction. (While you are reassuring the patient, also be sure that you have not missed unexpected LV dysfunction or aneurysm or silent ischemia.)

Return to Work and Disability Evaluation

Those in sedentary occupations are able to return to work 6 weeks after an uncomplicated MI. The average patient returns to work 2 to 3 months after MI. Those who do heavy physical work often need a longer period of rehabilitation. Uncertainty about a patient's ability to handle heavy work is an indication for exercise testing before returning to work. In some cases, it is a consideration when recommending angiography.

Your attitude and approach have a major influence on return to work. When the doctor outlines a timetable and exercise strategy aimed at return to work, the time off work is shortened. Earlier return has no adverse clinical effects, and there are financial and psychological advantages for the patient.

A number of patients seek medical disability after MI. In addition to cardiac symptoms, the Social Security Administration has objective criteria for awarding benefits, either depressed LVEF (below 30%) or evidence for ischemia on a stress test. Patients who do physical labor, have less education, or who are over 60 years old are less likely to return to work after MI.

Driving

A patient with a small uncomplicated MI may safely drive within 3 weeks of MI. I advise against long trips that early, suggesting short and nonstressful outings until later in recovery. The patient with large or complicated infarction is best advised to wait 6 weeks before starting to drive. It is wise to exclude arrhythmias and ischemia before agreeing to resumption of motor vehicle operation, using the risk stratification strategies described above.

SUGGESTED READINGS _____

Aldrich HR, Wagner B. Boswick J, et al. Use of initial ST-segment deviation for prediction of final electrocardiographic size of acute myocardial infarcts. Am J Cardiol 1988;61:749–753.

American Heart Association. Heart and Stroke Facts: 1998 Statistical Supplement. Dallas: American Heart Association, 1998.

Antman EM, Berlin JA. Declining incidence of ventricular fibrillation in myocardial infarction: implications for the prophylactic use of lidocaine. Circulation 1992;86:764–773.

Antman EM, Giugliano RP, Gibson CM, et al. Abciximab facilitates the rate and extent of thrombolysis: results of the TIMI 14 trial. Circulation 1999;99:2720–2732. (For a summary of other trials, see Califf RM. Glycoprotein IIb/IIIa blockade and thrombolytics; early lessons from the SPEED and Gusto IV trials. Am Heart J 1999;138:S12–S15.)

Barry WL, Sarembock IJ. Cardiogenic shock: therapy and prevention. Clin Cardiol 1998;21:72–80.

Buxton AE, Lee KL, Fisher JD, et al. A randomized study of the prevention of sudden death in patients with coronary artery disease. N Engl J Med 1999;341:1882–1890. (Results from 767 patients with LVEF < 40% and a history of MI who had inducible sustained ventricular tachycardia.)

Cardiac Arrhythmia Suppression Trial (CAST) Investigators. Preliminary report: effect of encainide and flecainide on mortality in a randomized trial of arrhythmia suppression after myocardial infarction. N Engl J Med 1989;321:406–412.

Dell'Italia LJ. Reperfusion for right ventricular infarction. N Engl J Med 1998;338:978–980.

Dennis C, Houston-Miller N, Schwartz RG, et al. Early return to work after uncomplicated myocardial infarction: results of a randomized trial. JAMA 1988;260:214–220.

Ewy GA, Appleton CP, Demaria AN, et al. ACC/AHA guidelines for the clinical application of echocardiography. A report of the American College of Cardiology/American Heart Association Task Force on Assessment of Diagnostic and Therapeutic Cardiovascular Procedures. J Am Coll Cardiol 1990;16:1505–1528.

Faxon DP, Heger JW. Primary angioplasty—enduring the test of time. N Engl J Med 1999;341:1464–1465.

Fibrinolytic Therapy Trialists' (FTT) Collaborative Group. Indications for fibrinolytic therapy in suspected acute myocardial infarction: collaborative overview of early mortality and major morbidity results from all randomized trials of more than 1000 patients. Lancet 1994;343:311–322.

Froelicher ES, Kee LL, Newton KM, et al. Return to work, sexual activity and other activities after acute myocardial infarction. Heart Lung 1994;23:423–435.

Galve E, Garcia-del-Castillo H, Evangelista A, et al. Pericardial effusion in the course of myocardial infarction: incidence, natural history, and clinical relevance. Circulation 1986;3:294–299.

Gheorghiade M, Bonow RO. Chronic heart failure in the United States: a manifestation of coronary artery disease. Circulation 1998;97:282–289.

Gibson RS, Boden WE, Theroux P, et al. Diltiazem and reinfarction in patients with non-Q wave myocardial infarction. N Engl J Med 1986;315:423–429.

Goldstein JA. Right heart ischemia: pathophysiology, natural history and clinical management. Prog Cardiovasc Disease 1998;40:325–341.

Guetta V, Topol EJ. Pacifying the infarct vessel. Circulation 1997;96:713–715.

The GUSTO Investigators. An international randomized trial comparing four thrombolytic strategies for acute myocardial infarction. N Engl J Med 1993;329:673–682.

Hamm CW, Goldmann BU, Heeschen C, et al. Emergency room triage of patients with acute chest pain by means of rapid testing for cardiac troponin T or troponin I. N Engl J Med 1997;337: 1648–1653.

Hennekens, CH, Albert CM, Godfried SL, et al. Adjunctive drug therapy of acute myocardial infarction: evidence from clinical trials. N Engl J Med 1996;335:1660–1667.

Higginbotham MB, Russell SD. Angiotensin II antagonists: present applications and future prospects in cardiovascular disease. Contemporary Int Med 1998;10:16–23.

Hochman, JS, Sleeper LA, Webb JG, et al. Early revascularization in acute myocardial infarction complicated by cardiogenic shock. The SHOCK trial. N Engl J Med 1999;341:625–634.

Honan MB, Harrell FE Jr, Reimer KA, et al. Cardiac rupture, mortality and the timing of thrombolytic therapy: a meta-analysis. J Am Coll Cardiol 1990;16:359–367.

ISIS-2 Collaborative Group. Randomized trial of intravenous streptokinase, oral aspirin, both, or neither among 17,187 cases of suspected acute myocardial infarction: ISIS-2. Lancet 1988;2: 349–360.

ISIS-4 Collaborative Group. ISIS-4: a randomized factorial trial assessing early oral captopril, oral mononitrate, and intravenous magnesium sulphate in 58,050 patients with suspected acute myocardial infarction. Lancet 1995;345:669–685.

Knoebel SB, Crawford MH, Dunn MI, et al. Guidelines for ambulatory electrocardiography. A report of the American College of Cardiology/American Heart Association Task Force on Assessment of Diagnostic and Therapeutic Cardiovascular Procedures. J Am Coll Cardiol 1989;13:249–258.

LATE Study Group. Late assessment of thrombolytic efficacy (LATE) study with alteplase 6–24 hours after onset of acute myocardial infarction. Lancet 1993;342:759–766.

Latini R, Maggioni AP, Flather M, et al. ACE-inhibitor use in patients with myocardial infarction: summary of evidence from clinical trials. Circulation 1995;92:3132–3137.

Lauer MA, Topol EJ. Taking the fibrinolytic era into the new millennium. Cardiol Rev 1999;16:10–20. (A good review of trials that combine lower dose rT-PA with aggressive antiplatelet therapy [glycoprotein IIb-IIIa receptor blockers].)

MacMahon S, Collins R, Peto R, et al. Effects of prophylactic lidocaine in suspected acute myocardial infarction: an overview of results from the randomized, controlled trials. JAMA 1988;260: 1910–1916.

Meijer A, Verheugt FWA, Werter CJPJ, et al. Aspirin versus Coumadin in the prevention of reocclusion and recurrent ischemia after successful thrombolysis: a prospective placebo-controlled angiographic study: results of the APRICOT study. Circulation 1993;68: 251–253.

Muller JE, Mittleman MA, Maclure M, et al. Triggering myocardial infarction by sexual activity. Low absolute risk and prevention by regular physical exertion. Determinants of Myocardial Infarction Onset Study Investigators. JAMA 1996;275:1405–1409.

O'Connor GT, Buring JE, Yusuf S, et al. An overview of randomized trials of rehabilitation with exercise after myocardial infarction. Circulation 1989;80:234–244.

Pepine CJ. Prognostic markers in thrombolytic therapy: looking beyond mortality. Am J Cardiol 1996;78(suppl 12A):24–27.

Peterson ED, Shaw LJ, Califf RM. Risk stratification after myocardial infarction. Ann Intern Med 1997;126:561–582.

Pratt CM, Waldo AL, Camm AJ. Can antiarrhythmic drugs survive the survival trials? Am J Cardiol 1998;81:24D–34D. (A review of all clinical trails of antiarrhythmic agents after MI, including the beta blocker trials.)

Reardon MJ, Carr CL, Diamond A, et al. Ischemic left ventricular free wall rupture: prediction, diagnosis and treatment. Ann Thorac Surg 1997;64:1509–1513.

Richard C, Ricome JL, Rimailho A, et al. Combined hemodynamic effects of dopamine and dobutamine in cardiogenic shock. Circulation 1983;67:620–626.

Ross J Jr, Brandenburg RO, Dinsmore RE, et al. Guidelines for coronary angiography. A report of the American College of Cardiology/American Heart Association Task Force on Assessment of Diagnostic and Therapeutic Cardiovascular Procedures. J Am Coll Cardiol 1987;10:935–950.

Ryan TJ, Anderson JL, Antman EM, et al. ACC/AHA Guidelines for the management of patients with acute myocardial infarction: executive summary. A report of the American College of Cardiology/American Heart Association Task Force on Practice Guidelines (Committee on Management of Acute Myocardial Infarction). Circulation 1996;94:2341–2350. (*Note update*: Ryan TJ, Antman EM, Brooks NH, et al. 1999 Update: ACC/AHA guidelines for the management of patients with acute myocardial infarction. J Am Coll Cardiol 1999;34:890–911.)

Scheidt S, Wilner G, Mueller H, et al. Intra-aortic balloon counterpulsation in cardiogenic shock: report of a cooperative clinical trial. N Engl J Med 1973;288:979–984.

Sgarbossa EB, Pinski SL, Barbagelata A, et al. Electrocardiographic diagnosis of evolving acute myocardial infarction in the presence of left bundle-branch block. N Engl J Med 1996;334: 481–487.

Silverman HW, Pfeifer MP. Relation between use of anti-inflammatory agents and left ventricular free wall rupture during acute myocardial infarction. Am J Cardiol 1987;59:363–364.

Simoons M, Maggioni A, Knatterud G, et al. Individual risk assessment for intracranial hemorrhage during thrombolytic therapy. Lancet 1993;342:1523–1528.

Simoons ML, Arnold AE. Tailored thrombolytic therapy: a perspective. Circulation 1993;88:2556–2564.

Stevenson R, Ranjadayalan K, Robert H, et al. Failure of post infarction exercise testing to predict coronary anatomy after thrombolysis: significance of reciprocal ST depression. J Am Coll Cardiol 1993;21:87A.

Taylor GJ, Katholi RE, Womack K, et al. Increased incidence of silent ischemia after acute myocardial infarction. JAMA 1992; 268:1448–1450. (In addition to demonstrating nociceptive dysfunction during induced ischemia, this study summarizes other clinical trials that demonstrate silent ischemia after reperfusion therapy.)

The TIMI Study Group. Comparison of invasive and conservative strategies after treatment with intravenous tissue plasminogen activator in acute myocardial infarction: results of the Thrombolysis in Myocardial Infarction (TIMI) Phase II Trial. N Engl J Med 1989; 320:618–627.

Tofler GH, Muller JA, Stone PH, et al. Pericarditis in acute myocardial infarction: characterization and clinical significance. Am Heart J 1989;117:86–90.

VanCamp SP, Peterson RA. Cardiovascular complications of outpatient cardiac rehabilitation programs. JAMA 1986;256:1160–1163.

Verstraete M. Third-generation thrombolytic drugs. Am J Med 2000;109:52–58. (Compared with rt-PA, newer drugs have improved early patency, but with no change in mortality; the risk of bleeding is higher.)

Weber KT. What can we learn from exercise testing beyond the detection of myocardial ischemia? Clin Cardiol 1997;20:684–696.

White HD, Barbash GI, Califf RM, et al. Age and outcome with contemporary thrombolytic therapy: results from the GUSTO–1 trial. Circulation 1996;94:1826–1833.

Yusef S, Peto R, Lewis J, et al. Beta blockade during and after myocardial infarction: an overview of the randomized trials. Prog Cardiovasc Dis 1985;27:335–371.

Yusuf S, Collins R, Lin L, et al. Significance of elevated MB isoenzyme with normal creatine kinase in acute myocardial infarction. Am J Cardiol 1987;59:245–250.

Zipes DP, DiMarco JP, Gillette PC, et al. Guidelines for clinical intracardiac electrophysiological studies and catheter ablation procedures. A report of the American College of Cardiology/American Heart Association Task Force on Practice Guidelines (Subcommittee to Assess Clinical Intracardiac Electrophysiological and Catheter Ablation Procedures). J Am Coll Cardiol 1995;26: 555–573.

CHAPTER 6

Cardiac Arrhythmias and Syncope

SUPRAVENTRICULAR ARRHYTHMIAS _____

Sinus Tachycardia, Bradycardia, and Sinus Arrhythmia

Whether or not *sinus tachycardia* (heart rate ≥ 100 beats/min) is a benign rhythm depends on the clinical setting. It is the normal response of a healthy person to exercise, excitement, or stress. It may point to noncardiac conditions such as anemia, thyrotoxicosis, or fever or may be caused by medicines (caffeine, amphetamines, thyroid hormone, or catecholamines).

Resting tachycardia in a person with heart disease usually indicates decompensation. The significance of this "arrhythmia" is often missed by inexperienced clinicians. Resting tachycardia a couple days after myocardial infarction (MI) is a marker of depressed left ventricular ejection fraction (LVEF). Although sinus tachycardia does not require specific treatment, it may be the only physical finding that indicates a bad prognosis. Interestingly, ventricular fibrillation (VF) during the first day of MI may occur with small infarction, where the long-term prognosis is good. Thus, persistent sinus tachycardia is a worse prognostic finding than VF at the onset of MI.

Sinus bradycardia, on the other hand, is usually an indicator of good cardiovascular fitness. It is common in trained athletes. Illnesses that cause bradycardia include hypothyroidism, sick sinus syndrome, and sleep apnea. Digitalis, β-adrenergic blockers, and the calcium channel blockers, verapamil and diltiazem, also cause sinus slowing. On the other hand, the dihydropyridine class of calcium blockers are pure vasodilators with no direct effect on the sinus node, and there is usually reflex tachycardia (nifedipine, amlodipine, felodipine).

Sinus arrhythmia is a common variant that should not be considered an arrhythmia, because it reflects normal cardiac function. Recall how heart rate is controlled by the autonomic nervous system. Increased sympathetic tone raises the rate, a reflex response to increased demand that happens over a period of seconds; withdrawal of sympathetic tone leads to a fall in rate, also over a period of seconds.

Sinus arrhythmia is a more rapid, beat-to-beat variation in rate. You see variation in the RR interval on the electrocardiogram (ECG) (and may see a healthy young person in cardiology clinic with "irregular heart beat"). It is a vagal rather than a sympathetic phenomenon. With inspiration and increased venous return to the heart, stroke volume rises. The vagus is activated, and heart rate slows temporarily, with no change in cardiac output (cardiac output = heart rate × stroke volume). During expiration there is a decrease in venous return to the chest and heart, and withdrawal of vagal tone leads to a temporary increase in heart rate.

The normal response to poor LV function and reduced cardiac output is to shut down the parasympathetic system and to increase sympathetic tone. There is no respiratory variation in vagal output, and the heart rate becomes quite regular. The absence of sinus arrhythmia is thus a marker of LV dysfunction. This concept has been found clinically useful after MI, because a loss of heart rate variability may be measured and is a predictor of low LVEF and bad prognosis (see Table 5.13).

Premature Atrial Contractions

Premature atrial contractions (PACs) are usually easy to recognize (Fig. 6.1). The QRS complex is narrow, as the right and left ventricles depolarize simultaneously. The QRS of the premature beat looks like the normal sinus beats. There may be an ectopic misshapen P wave before it, occasionally buried in the preceding T wave.

A *blocked PAC* may be the cause of a pause on the ECG and may be felt by the patient as a "skipped beat." This happens when the PAC is early enough that the atrioventricular (AV) node is refractory and will not conduct it. The ectopic P wave may be buried in the preceding T wave, making it easy to miss. Look for alteration of the T wave just before the pause when you see this on the board exam (Fig. 6.1).

PACs are common in healthy people and do not indicate heart disease. If the ECG, cardiac history, and examination are normal, no further testing or treatment is necessary.

Paroxysmal Supraventricular Tachycardia

Paroxysmal supraventricular tachycardia (PSVT) is a rapid regular rhythm with a rate of 120 to 200 beats/min. Most cases are caused by reentry within the AV node. Reentry is a common mechanism of both atrial and ventricular tachyarrhythmias. Although frequently misunderstood, the concept is fairly simple (Fig. 6.2). The reentrant focus is a region that is protected, or insulated, from surrounding tissue. Current enters one end of the focus and exits the other (conduction is unidirectional). Within the reentrant focus, conduction is much slower than conduction through surrounding tissue. By the time current exits the focus, the surrounding tissue has depolarized and has had time to recover. Thus, the current exiting the focus finds the surrounding tissue vulnerable and ready to be stimulated. That is just what happens, and a premature beat is generated. A reentrant focus in the atrium causes a PAC, and a reentrant focus in the body of the ventricle causes a premature ventricular contraction (PVC).

If the timing is perfect, the premature beat may slip back into the entrance of the reentrant focus, leading to another or even to a series of ectopic beats, usually at a rapid rate. A "reentrant circuit" is created.

AV nodal reentry is the usual mechanism of PSVT. Current exiting the focus passes normally through the common His bundle, and the resulting QRS complex is narrow (again, the sequence of ventricular activation is normal with simultaneous right ventricular and LV depolarization). PSVT is therefore a "narrow complex tachycardia" (Fig. 6.3). There are two exceptions to this general rule. First, a patient may have coexisting bundle branch block. Second, a diseased infranodal conduction system may be stressed by the fast heart rate, and there is "aberrant conduction," most commonly right bundle branch block. The right bundle tends to be the weakest link in the conduction system, the

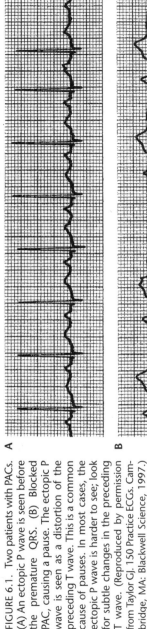

FIGURE 6.1. Two patients with PACs. (A) An ectopic P wave is seen before the premature QRS. (B) Blocked PAC, causing a pause. The ectopic P wave is seen as a distortion of the preceding T wave. This is a common cause of pauses. In most cases, the ectopic P wave is harder to see; look for subtle changes in the preceding T wave. (Reproduced by permission from Taylor GJ. 150 Practice ECGs. Cambridge, MA: Blackwell Science, 1997.)

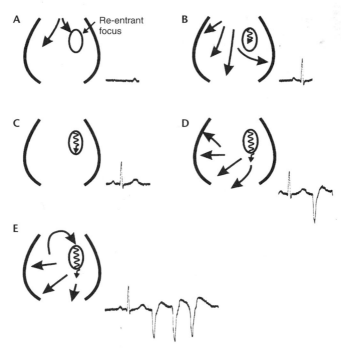

FIGURE 6.2. Reentry. Follow the sequence of events. (A) The wave of depolarization comes from above (the atrium in the case of atrial arrhythmias, the ventricle in this case of ventricular reentry). (B) As current moves through the myocardium, it also enters the reentrant focus, a region that is insulated from the surrounding tissue. (C) Depolarization of the surrounding myocardium happens quickly, but conduction through the reentrant focus is slow. (D) By the time current exits the reentrant focus, the surrounding tissue has been repolarized and is *vulnerable*. That is to say, it can be stimulated. This produces the *ectopic beat*. (E) If the timing is perfect, current from the ectopic beat reenters the protected focus, travels through it, and again finds the surrounding tissue vulnerable when it exits. A circuit is established and the result is repetitive ectopic beats. Characteristics of the reentrant focus that make this possible: insulation from surrounding tissue, unidirectional conduction, and slow conduction. (Reproduced by permission from Taylor GJ. 150 Practice ECGs. Cambridge, MA: Blackwell Science, 1997.)

first to fail at high heart rates. Right bundle branch block is a clue that a wide complex tachycardia is SVT with aberrancy rather than ventricular tachycardia (VT).

PSVT is a common arrhythmia in otherwise healthy young people. It is not dangerous, but it can be bothersome, causing

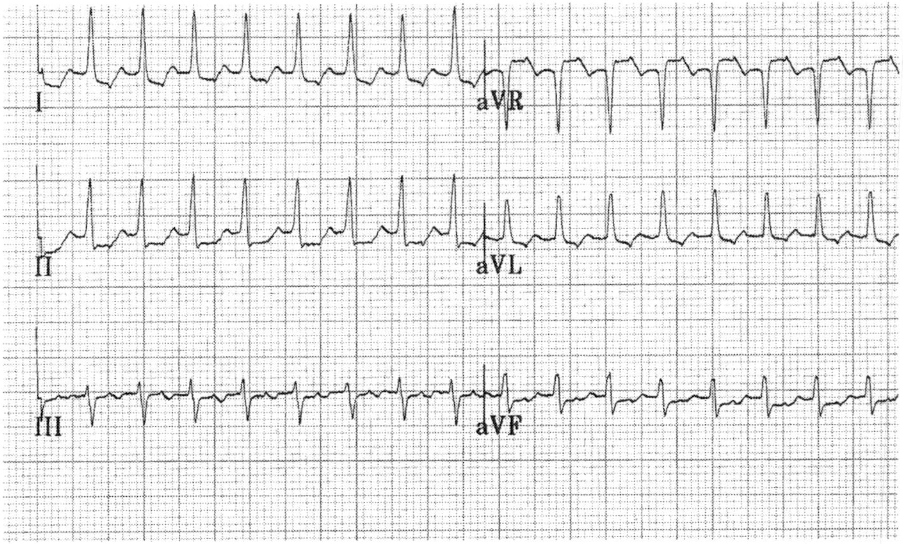

FIGURE 6.3. PSVT, a recording of limb leads. The rate is 200 beats/min. The T waves appear distorted, and these distortions may be ectopic P waves. This episode lasted 45 min, plenty of time to get an ECG. (Reproduced by permission from Taylor GJ. 150 Practice ECGs. Cambridge, MA: Blackwell Science, 1997.)

palpitations, dizziness, and near-syncope. It is uncommon to have loss of consciousness. Drugs that slow AV node conduction may control symptoms (beta-blockers, digoxin, verapamil, or diltiazem), and intravenous adenosine may interrupt the tachycardia. When symptoms are frequent and not easily controlled, *radiofrequency ablation* of the reentrant focus is possible using catheter techniques. Many patients find this cure preferable to life-long drug therapy.

Electrophysiology (EP) testing is needed to "map" the site of reentry. Box 6.1 summarizes the uses of EP testing (page 231).

Preexcitation

Preexcitation, including the Wolff-Parkinson-White syndrome, is the archetypal reentrant rhythm and is a favorite of board examiners. The mechanism of the arrhythmia is described in Figure 6.4. Normally, there is a layer of connective tissue separating the atria and ventricles that serves as insulation, preventing free passage of neural impulses between the upper and lower chambers. The AV node is the normal passage through this layer of insulation. Slow conduction through the AV node allows time for atrial systole to complete ventricular filling before ventricular systole. The preexcitation syndrome occurs because of an additional "defect" in the insulation between atria and ventricles. This defect is called a *bypass tract*. As the wave of depolarization passes through the atria, it leaks through the bypass tract and into the AV node.

Conduction through the bypass tract usually is faster than AV node conduction. As current exits the bypass tract, it stimulates the ventricle; it is "preexcited." An instant later, current exits the AV node and also stimulates the ventricle. The ventricular complex originating from two sites is a "fusion beat." The QRS is wider than normal and starts earlier after the P wave, so the PR interval appears to be short. The initial slurred portion of the QRS caused by preexcitation of the ventricle through the bypass tract is the delta wave (Fig. 6.4).

The bypass tract can conduct either antegrade or retrograde. A premature atrial beat that finds the accessory pathway refractory may pass through the AV node, capture the ventricle, conduct retrograde through the accessory pathway, and establish a reentrant circuit. Because antegrade conduction is through the AV node, the reentrant arrhythmia looks like SVT with a narrow

Preexcitation of the Left Ventricle Through a Bypass Tract

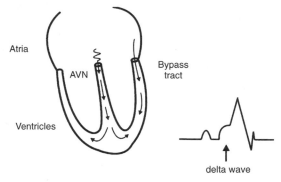

delta wave

Two patterns of supraventricular tachycardia

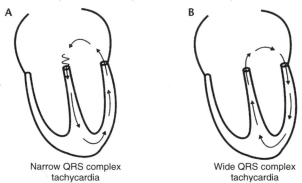

Narrow QRS complex
tachycardia

Wide QRS complex
tachycardia

FIGURE 6.4. Preexcitation (or the Wolff-Parkinson-White syndrome). This cartoon illustrates the changes caused by a bypass tract between the atria and ventricles. The tract is located on the LV side and near the mitral valve in this particular patient, but bypass tracts may be located at any site where atria and ventricles come into contact. Simultaneous activation of the ventricles via the bypass tract and the AV node produce a fusion beat. Conduction through the bypass tract is faster than through the AV node. Early activation of the ventricle produces the delta wave and makes the PR interval appear short.

A reentrant circuit can develop between the bypass tract and the AV node, resulting in supraventricular tachycardia. There are two possibilities. A: The reentrant circuit moves antegrade through the AV node, retrograde through the bypass tract. The sequence of ventricular activation is therefore normal, and the QRS is narrow. B: The reentrant circuit is directed retrograde through the AV node and antegrade through the bypass tract. Because activation of the ventricles originates from the lateral wall of the LV, the QRS complex is wide. (Reproduced by permission from Taylor GJ. 150 Practice ECGs. Cambridge, MA: Blackwell Science, 1997.)

QRS complex. A reentrant circuit in the opposite direction, retrograde through the AV node and antegrade through the accessory pathway, and produces a wide QRS complex because the sequence of ventricular activation is abnormal. The resulting wide complex tachycardia looks like VT.

How can you tell whether the wide complex tachycardia is ventricular or supraventricular? At times you cannot, just from the ECG. The clinical setting helps. A young patient with a history of PSVT, no prior heart disease, and little alteration of consciousness is more likely to have PSVT with bypass tract reentry. An older patient with syncope or near-syncope plus a history of heart failure or MI should be treated assuming a diagnosis of VT. When in doubt, it is hard to go wrong treating an *unstable* patient with wide complex tachycardia as probable VT. Direct current (DC) cardioversion is appropriate.

It is important to identify PSVT that is caused by preexcitation because the medical therapy is different. Digoxin should be avoided because it shortens the refractory period of the accessory pathway and blocks the AV node. If the patient has atrial flutter or fibrillation, these actions may favor antegrade conduction through the accessory pathway and an unusually rapid ventricular rate. Verapamil and lidocaine may also accelerate the ventricular response with atrial fibrillation (AF) or flutter. By contrast, membrane active antiarrhythmic agents slow accessory pathway conduction; intravenous procainamide is a safe choice.

Membrane active drugs have been used for long-term management as well. However, catheter ablation of the accessory pathway usually works and is preferable to life-long drug therapy. Radiofrequency energy is delivered to the area of the bypass tract, burns it (about like a sunburn), and the resulting scar tissue plugs the defect in the insulation.

Nodal (Junctional) Rhythm

It is recognized by the absence of P waves before the QRS, and the rhythm is regular (Fig. 6.5). Although tachycardia (rate ≥ 100 beats/min) is possible, the heart rate is usually within the normal range. Stimulation of the ventricles comes from the AV node, so the QRS complex is narrow (unless there is preexisting bundle branch block). There may be retrograde depolarization of the

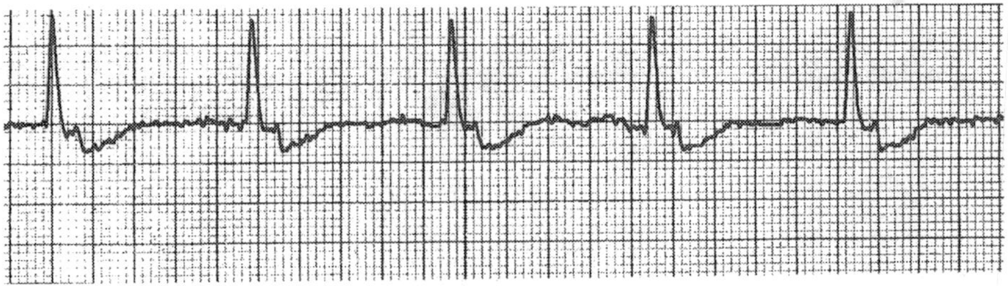

FIGURE 6.5. Nodal (or *junctional*) rhythm. The retrograde P wave distorting the T wave is prominent in this example. Usually it is more subtle, and it may be absent. Even without retrograde P waves, the diagnosis of junctional rhythm may be made when the rate is regular, is less than 100 beats/min, and there are no P waves. The QRS is usually narrow. (Reproduced by permission from Taylor GJ. 150 Practice ECGs. Cambridge, MA: Blackwell Science, 1997.)

atria, and retrograde P waves may fall within and distort either the QRS complex or the T wave (Fig. 6.5).

Nodal rhythm is not dangerous and requires no specific therapy. It may be a marker of digitalis toxicity. Nodal and other atrial tachyarrhythmias that occur in a setting of recent MI are more common with large infarction and LV dysfunction.

Atrial Fibrillation (AF) and Flutter

AF is the most common arrhythmia requiring treatment in hospitalized patients. It may paroxysmal or chronic. Patients with structurally normal hearts by echocardiogram may experience AF with electrolyte abnormalities (commonly low potassium or magnesium), alcohol intoxication (the "holiday heart" syndrome), or thyrotoxicosis. Recurrent paroxysmal AF may be idiopathic, although many with this condition have a history of hypertension, raising the possibility of elevated left atrial pressure.

Both AF and flutter are reentrant rhythms. The flutter circuit is at the base of the right atrium, between the tricuspid valve and the inferior vena cava (with chronic flutter ablation is a possibility). The reentrant circuit in AF is more diffuse, with most of it in the left atrium. A major difference between the two rhythms is the atrial rate; with flutter it is predictably at 300 beats/min and with AF it is considerably faster, as high as 600 beats/min.

Recognition of these arrhythmias is straightforward. AF is irregular, and flutter is regular with a saw-toothed P wave pattern (Fig. 6.6). The flutter waves may not be apparent with just one ECG lead. Think of it when there is a regular rhythm at 150 beats/min and confirm the diagnosis with a 12-lead ECG. The occasional patient who does not have obvious flutter waves on a surface ECG may require an ECG lead closer to the atria, either a right atrial or esophageal electrode. With either electrode system the P waves are larger and thus visible.

New atrial flutter in an elderly bedridden patient may be an early sign of pulmonary embolus. One of my teachers suggested thinking of atrial flutter as a rhythm originating from the right atrium and AF as a left atrial arrhythmia. This is simplistic, and there is enough overlap that the concept cannot be generalized. Nevertheless, it is interesting that flutter often complicates pulmonary problems such as obstructive lung disease and pulmonary embolus (see Chapter 7 for discussion of cor pulmonale).

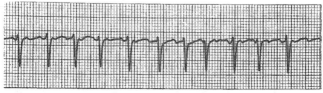

A

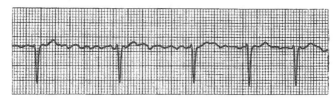

B

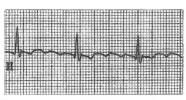

C

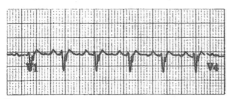

D

FIGURE 6.6. Four patients with SVT. (A) AF with rapid ventricular response; at higher rates, the variation in the RR interval seen with AF may be subtle. (B) AF with a controlled ventricular response; with drug therapy to slow AV node conduction, the ventricular rate is kept between 80 and 100 beats/min. In this case, you can see the fibrillation waves as coarse undulation in the baseline. (C) Atrial flutter with 2:1 block; note the sawtooth pattern in the baseline. (D) Atrial flutter with 4:1 block; the flutter waves are more obvious. (Reproduced by permission from Taylor GJ. 150 Practice ECGs. Cambridge, MA: Blackwell Science, 1997.)

AF, on the other hand, is a common complication of hypertension and mitral valve disease (left heart illnesses).

AF usually causes palpitations. Loss of atrial contraction also results in an abrupt fall in cardiac output (see Figure 1.8), and the

TABLE 6.1. Management of AF and Flutter

Therapy	Comment
Ventricular rate control	Drugs that slow AV node conduction: digoxin, beta-blockers, diltiazem, and verapamil. Those with normal AV node function often need two drugs for control.
Anticoagulation— warfarin*	All patients with structural heart disease (valvular disease, depressed LV function, marked LA enlargement), and all ≥ 65 years old. Target INR = 2–2.5 (with a prosthetic valve or prior thromboembolism, 3–3.5).
Anticoagulation— aspirin 325 mg/day	Young people (<60 years old) with normal LV function, no structural changes on the echocardiogram, and no history of thromboemboli. Others with contraindications to warfarin therapy.
Urgent DC cardioversion	Any patient with a rapid supraventricular rhythm and hemodynamic instability or ongoing angina. *Do not waste time pushing rate-lowering drugs when the patient is unstable.*
Elective DC cardioversion	May be considered for any patient, but it is unlikely to work with marked LA enlargement or chronic AF (more than 3 months). Cardioversion is safe without anticoagulation within 48 hours of the onset of AF; after that, anticoagulate and cardiovert 3–4 weeks later.
Medical cardioversion	Ibutilide works in about half the cases, and it improves the results with DC cardioversion. Give 1 mg, wait 10 minutes, and give a second dose. Proceed with DC cardioversion 20–30 minutes later.
Maintaining sinus rhythm	*Normal LV function:* sotalol, flecainide or propafenone. *Depressed LV function:* amiodarone (first choice, though quinidine and procainamide are alternatives). See Table 6.5. These drugs may also be used for cardioversion.

*The risk of thromboembolism is lower with chronic atrial flutter than it is with AF. However, there still is risk, and anticoagulation is indicated. LA, left atrium; INR, International Normalized Ratio (preferable to the prothrombin time).

patient may complain of weakness or loss of energy. This is more common when there is LV diastolic dysfunction (see Chapter 1). There may be dizziness, but syncope is rare.

Treatment of AF and Atrial Flutter

Rate Control When the patient is hemodynamically stable, the first task is control of the ventricular rate (Table 6.1). All the AV nodal blocking drugs are effective, and your first choice may be influenced by other heart conditions. For example, if there is low LVEF, digoxin might be a better choice than verapamil or beta-blockers, as both depress LV contractility. On the other hand, these drugs would be good for the patient with hyperdynamic LV contractility and LV hypertrophy. It is common to need two different drugs to control the rate when it is especially rapid. A heart rate below 100 beats/min indicates underlying AV node disease, and medical therapy to further block the AV node is unnecessary. Atrial flutter with 3:1 block and a stable rate of 100 beats/min may be treated with an AV node blocking drug to prevent increases in rate (more rapid AV node conduction) with exercise.

A common mistake with digoxin therapy is inadequate dosing. The digoxin level should not be used to place a ceiling on the dose; even if the level is high, you may titrate the dose to the ventricular rate. In practice, we more commonly treat with digoxin 0.25 mg/day and then add a second AV node blocking drug (diltiazem, verapamil, or a beta-blocker) to reel the heart rate in. That way other features of digitalis toxicity are more easily avoided (nausea, anorexia, visual changes, and other arrhyhthmias). Symptoms of digitalis toxicity may be subtle, are often overlooked in older patients, and may occur when the digoxin level is in the therapeutic range.

The Unstable Patient A common management error is the failure to cardiovert the patient who is hemodynamically unstable because of the rapid heart rate. Severe hypotension and other clinical evidence for shock may develop with new AF when there is diastolic dysfunction, especially in the case of critical aortic valve stenosis (review the discussion of diastolic dysfunction and preload dependence in Chapter 1). Coronary artery disease and intractable angina with new-onset rapid AF should also be considered unstable. In such cases it is a mistake and a waste of time to push medicines to reduce the ventricular rate, because medicine loading usually requires repetitive dosing over a period of hours.

This is a medical emergency. If it is your judgment that the patient is unstable because of the tachyarrhythmia, emergency DC cardioversion is the proper treatment (vide infra).

Anticoagulation When I talk with patients with AF, I emphasize that the arrhythmia itself is not dangerous. I have patients who have done well with AF for decades. Morbidity and mortality are usually the result of embolic stroke. The risk of stroke in subsets of patients with AF is as follows:

- Rheumatic heart disease (mitral stenosis)—a 17-fold increase, an 8% per year risk of stroke;
- AF without mitral stenosis—4% per year risk of stroke;

- Patients less than 60 years old and a normal echocardiogram—1% per year risk of stroke.

There is an intermediate risk of stroke with a normal mitral valve but an abnormal echocardiogram, including a dilated and poorly functioning left ventricle or a severely dilated left atrium. On the other hand, a young person with a normal echo has a low, but not a zero, risk.

Based on these natural history data plus randomized clinical trials, anticoagulation using warfarin is recommended for patients with AF and an abnormal echocardiogram and for all patients older than 65 years (Table 6.1). This reduces the risk of peripheral embolization by almost 75% when the International Normalization Ratio is maintained between 2.0 and 3.0. Although not supported by clinical trials, it is common practice to treat low-risk young patients with "lone AF" (i.e., a normal echocardiogram) with aspirin.

Contraindications to warfarin include recent stroke, uncontrolled hypertension, recent surgery or bleeding, and medical noncompliance. In such cases, aspirin 325 mg/day may be substituted. Although not as effective as warfarin, it has been shown to reduce the incidence of embolization by 44%.

Chronic atrial flutter increases the risk of thromboembolism, but not as much as AF. When there is no contraindication, follow the AF guidelines for anticoagulation.

Cardioversion Brief duration of AF and a normal-sized left atrium are predictors of success with either medical or DC cardioversion. It is probably not worth the effort and discomfort for the patient who has been in AF for 4 to 6 months or more, although late cardioversion is occasionally attempted when there is heart failure due to diastolic dysfunction (see Chapter 1).

Post operative AF is a common in-hospital consultation. It is often caused by low potassium or magnesium and converts with electrolyte replacement. *Hypomagnesemia* is frequently overlooked. Push the magnesium level to more than 2.2 mEq/L. This usually requires 6 to 10 g $MgSO_4$ given intravenously (I give it in two doses separated by an hour, with each infused over 20 minutes). Hypomagnesemia may be caused by diuretics. Anything that lowers potassium also lowers magnesium. Oral magnesium replacement is often ineffective, because Mg^{+2} ion is poorly absorbed (which is why it is a good laxative). It turns out that the potassium-sparing diuretic spironolactone also raises serum magnesium and is an effective long-term treatment; in one trial 50 mg spironolactone per day raised the serum Mg^{2+} by 13% (see Chapter 1).

Ibutilide is particularly effective for new-onset AF or flutter in the hospital (Table 6.1). It may also be used in conjunction with DC cardioversion for more established AF and increases the chance for success. A logistically neat approach is ibutilide infusion and then DC cardioversion a half-hour later if AF has not converted.

DC cardioversion is technically simple. Set the machine to the synchronized mode so that the shock is delivered well after the T wave. Use plenty of electrode jelly and ensure firm contact with the chest wall to avoid burning the skin. Correct electrode position is needed to deliver current across the heart. Both anterior-posterior electrodes and mid-chest-lateral-chest positions work, though the former is currently favored. DC shock hurts, and we have an anesthetist push drugs. In an urgent situation, give Versed 1–2 mg intravenously in repeated doses until the patient is unable to count backward.

Atrial flutter is sensitive to DC shock, and conversion may occur with as little as 10 to 15 J. To avoid repeated shocks I usually start with 50 J, because this works for most patients. It is common for flutter to convert to AF with DC shock; if this happens, proceed with repeat shock to convert the AF.

AF is more resistant to DC shock. Begin with 200 J, but you will usually need maximum output to convert (360 to 400 J).

Anticoagulation and Cardioversion If the patient has been in AF or flutter for less than 48 hours, you may cardiovert without anticoagulation. After 48 hours, start warfarin, wait at least 3 weeks, and cardiovert electively. The risk of peripheral embolization persists after restoration of sinus rhythm, and warfarin should be continued for 6 weeks. Brief-duration AF does not require anticoagulation after cardioversion, though I commonly prescribe aspirin.

Hospital Admission and Telemetry During Cardioversion The risk of provoking ventricular arrhythmias (VAs) is low with class IC drugs when LV function is normal, but it is not zero. Proarrhythmia is dose dependent with these agents and is apt to occur late after starting treatment. Nevertheless, our electrophysiology (EP) service usually admits the patient for 3 days when chemical cardioversion is attempted with flecainide or propafenone. If AF persists, then DC cardioversion, with or without ibutilide, is done on the third day.

Maintaining Sinus Rhythm Drugs that slow AV conduction, such as digoxin, beta-blockers, and calcium channel blockers, are no more effective than placebo for cardioversion. Nor do they prevent recurrence of AF or flutter after cardioversion.

Postoperative short-duration AF seldom recurs, and I do not routinely send patients home with antiarrhythmic drug therapy. If antiarrhythmic drugs have been prescribed, they may be stopped in 1 month.

In other clinical situations, AF is more likely to recur after cardioversion. I usually treat the patient with a membrane-active agent for 3 to 6 months and then stop it (Table 6.1). I do not commit the patient to life-long antiarrhythmic therapy unless there is subsequent recurrence of AF.

Invasive Therapy for AF and Flutter Catheter ablation for atrial flutter is now possible. A line of scar from the tricuspid annulus to the inferior vena cava may interrupt the reentrant circuit. Similar techniques for AF have not been as successful, because the reentrant circuit involves a large portion of the left atrium. The Maze operation may work, with extensive incisions in both atria, but morbidity and mortality have been high.

Catheter ablation of the AV node has been more useful and should be considered when rate control is difficult with chronic AF. A permanent pacemaker is inserted, and a couple weeks later the AV node is ablated. The patient no longer needs rate-lowering drugs, avoiding their side effects. Although unproved, there is speculation that a more regular rhythm may improve overall cardiac function for some patients, and the ventricular pacemaker provides that.

For a brief period after AV node ablation, there is an increased risk of sudden death. This has been attributed to the slower heart rate leading to lower threshold for torsade de pointes (see below). To avoid this complication, the pacemaker is initially set at 90 beats/min, and the rate is cut back a few months later.

Automatic Ectopic Tachycardia

Most atrial tachyarrhythmias are reentrant. It is possible to have enhanced automaticity of pacemaker fibers as a cause of SVT.

Atrial ectopic tachycardia is rare, with a rate of 140 to 160 beats/min. For this reason it may be confused with atrial flutter. It usually is sustained, tends to resist medical therapy, and is diagnosed with an electrophysiology study (EPS). The most effective treatment is catheter ablation of the automatic focus. Some cases of junctional tachycardia come from an automatic focus in the AV node, and there may be retrograde P waves (Fig. 6.5). The most effective drugs to suppress automaticity are beta-blockers, calcium channel blockers, and amiodarone.

Multifocal atrial tachycardia is a more common automatic atrial rhythm. The usual clinical setting is poorly compensated obstructive lung disease. It is an irregular rhythm and may be confused with AF on physical exam. The ECG shows definite P waves before each QRS complex (i.e., there is no AV dissociation) but with variation in P wave morphology. When the rate is above 100 beats/min it is called multifocal atrial tachycardia; at lower rates it may be called wandering atrial pacemaker (Fig. 6.7). The best treatment is improving pulmonary function. Verapamil or diltiazem may slow the rate; digoxin and other antiarrhythmic drugs usually do not help. It is unusual for the rate to be so fast that cardiac function is compromised.

Tachycardia-induced Cardiomyopathy

This may occur with a sustained atrial tachyarrhythmia. A typical case is the patient with rapid AF and symptoms of heart failure who is found to have depressed LV function on the echocardiogram. The patient may be able to point to a change in exercise tolerance a month or so earlier, indicating the onset of the arrhythmia. With control of ventricular rate, EF and symptoms improve over the next few months. In such cases, afterload reduction therapy for heart failure is also important, and I usually continue it for 6 to 12 months after LV function has improved (although no clinical trials data guide the duration of therapy).

VENTRICULAR ARRHYTHMIAS

Etiology of Complex VAs and the Risk of Sudden Death

The clinical setting determines the prognosis with VAs. PVCs may be considered a normal variant in the healthy patient

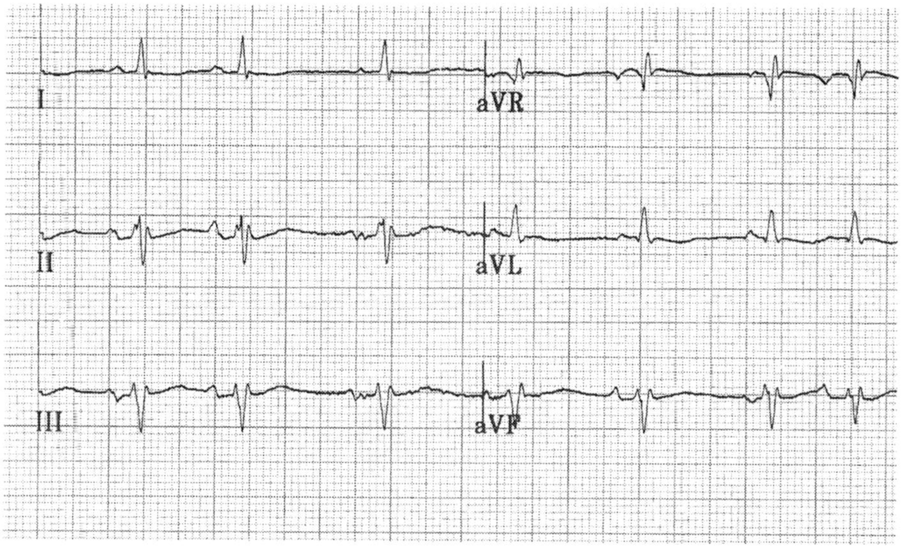

FIGURE 6.7. Wandering atrial pacemaker. These limb leads are from a patient with obstructive lung disease. The variation in P wave morphology is seen in lead II. Note the variable rate (RR interval). In the absence of obvious P waves before each QRS, this would look like atrial fibrillation. At rates above 100 beats/min, wandering atrial pacemaker becomes MAT. (Reproduced by permission from Taylor GJ. 150 Practice ECGs. Cambridge, MA: Blackwell Science, 1997.)

TABLE 6.2. VAs, a Hierarchy of RISK*

Isolated PVC	A normal finding in healthy people, and the prognosis is good if the echocardiogram is normal. Hard to suppress with antiarrhythmic therapy; you may try beta blockade if the patient is symptomatic.
Complex VAs (multifocal PVCs or pairs)	More common with depressed LV function. Not an indication for therapy, but if the patient is symptomatic, try a beta-blocker. The risk of sudden cardiac death (SCD) is increased if LVEF is low. Syncope or near-syncope raises the possibility of VT. Be sure that potassium and magnesium are normal.
VT	As above, and a much higher risk for SCD. Sustained VT is the usual indication for implantable defibrillator therapy. "Nonsustained" VT = 3 or more sequential PVCs < s30 seconds in duration. "Sustained" VT is >30 seconds in duration.
Torsade de pointes	A complication of QT interval prolongation (see Table 5.7) and often occurs with normal LV function. The prognosis is good if the QT interval can be normalized.
Accelerated idioventricular rhythm	An automatic rather than reentrant rhythm. It occurs frequently when coronary perfusion is reestablished during acute MI. Short lived. Not a marker of poor LV function. It seldom degenerates to VF, and is resistant to drug therapy.

*This table does not consider VT or VF during the acute phase of MI. Acute-phase VT and VF are not closely linked to LV function and may complicate a small MI. Assuming successful treatment of the arrhythmia, they do not indicate bad prognosis.

with a structurally normal heart and normal LV function (Table 6.2).

During the acute phase of MI, complex VAs, including VT and VF, may occur with just minimal LV injury; the reentrant arrhythmia is a purely electrical event. But later after MI, complex VAs are associated with severe LV dysfunction and thus indicate poor prognosis. The evaluation and treatment of VAs after MI—which applies to all with ischemic heart disease—are reviewed in Chapter 5. Of special interest are the findings of the Cardiac Arrhythmia Suppression Trial (CAST), which discovered that the proarrhythmic effects of membrane-active antiarrhythmic drugs overshadow any beneficial effects (see Table 5.11). Although this was a study of patients with prior MI and LV dysfunction, the results have been applied to most with complex VAs, and we no longer "chase PVCs" with antiarrhythmic therapy.

Pathophysiology of VAs

Isolated PVCs may come from either an automatic focus or a reentrant focus (Fig. 6.2). Repetitive ventricular ectopics, with three or more in a row defined as VT, are usually reentrant. That is certainly the case with VF.

A prominent exception is accelerated idioventricular rhythm, often called "slow VT." The rate may be less than 100 beats/min, and the ectopic focus works like a fixed rate pacemaker. When the sinus rate falls below the ectopic rate, it "takes over" and paces the heart until the intrinsic rate increases. This rhythm is common at the time of reperfusion during thrombolytic therapy for MI (and has been proposed as a marker of reperfusion). It is considered benign, because it rarely degenerates to VF; drug therapy (lidocaine) usually does not suppress it.

VAs are aggravated by *low potassium or magnesium*. Sudden cardiac death is caused by VF. Community-based studies have found that sudden cardiac death is more frequent with diuretic therapy and that survivors often have hypokalemia. These patients invariably have other heart disease and LV dysfunction as well, but the electrolyte abnormality is the final straw. The first thing I do with all "rhythm consults" is check electrolytes, an easy thing to fix. Plus, if you do not fix electrolyte abnormalities, the arrhythmia will be tough to control. Do not overlook magnesium; like potassium, it falls with diuresis and is also low after surgery or trauma.

Laboratory Diagnosis
Noninvasive Testing

Ventricular ectopics have a wide QRS complex that is distorted and has a different axis than normal complexes. At times there is uncertainty about whether ectopic beats are ventricular or atrial with aberrant conduction, and criteria that help with the diagnosis are in Table 6.3.

The workup of the patient with palpitations is fairly simple (Table 6.4). *Evaluating LV function* is as important as identifying arrhythmias with ECG monitoring, because normal function excludes complex ventricular ectopy for practical purposes. We used to do a lot of 24-hour (Holter) monitoring, back when we chased PVCs with drug therapy. Serial monitors were done to test the effectiveness of treatment. Now I use the 24-hour monitor to evaluate symptoms, usually syncope or near-syncope. Occasionally I order one to diagnose VT in a patient with coronary

TABLE 6.3. Differentiating a PVC from an Aberrantly Conducted Supraventricular Ectopic Beat (or Distinguishing VT from SVT With Aberrant Conduction)

Favors PVC or VT	Favors Supraventricular Beat or SVT
In precordial leads, the complexes are monophasic (no biphasic, RS complexes). The T wave axis is usually opposite the QRS axis (it is not "concordant")	Aberrant conduction often causes a right bundle branch block (RBBB) pattern, with a triphasic, RSR complex in V_1
AV dissociation proves VT	A P wave linked to every QRS complex proves SVT
QRS in V_1 is positive (as with RBBB) but is also monomorphic	
Very wide QRS (the onset of the R wave to the deepest part of the S wave > 100 msec in multiple leads)	

TABLE 6.4. Workup of Palpitations

Test	Comment
ECG	1. Narrow QRS, infranodal heart block unlikely.
	2. Q waves (and a history of MI) increase the chance of low LVEF and VAs.
	3. Short PR and delta wave, preexcitation syndromes.
	4. Long QT interval, increased risk of VAs, see Table 6.7
Electrolytes	Low magnesium or potassium increase the risk of both VA and supraventricular arrhythmia. Note a history of diuretic use.
Echocardiogram	1. VAs usually occur in patients with depressed LV function, and normal LVEF rules out VT (with rare exceptions, see Table 6.6). There is no need to pursue further monitoring for complex VAs as part of the initial screen.
	2. Left atrial size determines the prognosis for successful medical control of AF, and the absence of structural abnormalities indicates a lower risk of thromboembolism.
24-Hour (Holter) monitor	Complex VAs are always there, and you will not miss them with a single 24-hour monitor. Supraventricular arrhythmias often are intermittent and may be missed with just one day of monitoring.
Event monitor	The patient has the monitor for weeks, and activates it when there are symptoms. This is best for detecting intermittent supraventricular arrhythmias (e.g., paroxysmal AF). It is especially useful for excluding arrhythmias as a cause of "palpitations."
EPS	1. Bradyarrhythmias: to determine the level of AV block.
	2. VAs: EPS is reserved for the patient with suspected VT as the cause of syncope based on screening studies.
Testing for coronary artery disease	Reserved for patients with symptomatic and complex VAs (usually with low LVEF). In the absence of suggestive symptoms, an abnormal ECG or regional wall motion abnormalities on echo, noninvasive screening is ok.

artery disease and depressed LVEF. Other noninvasive tests that show an increased risk of VT and are markers of low LVEF in patients with prior MI are heart rate variability and the signal-averaged ECG (Table 5.13).

The diagnosis of coronary artery disease is usually obvious from the history and ECG. When the diagnosis of coronary artery disease is uncertain, it is important to screen for it with either a perfusion scan (when the probability seems remote) or coronary angiography (when coronary artery disease seems more likely). Revascularization may be an important element of treatment when there is active ischemia.

Electrophysiology (EP) Testing

In the catheterization laboratory, one or more electrode catheters are positioned in the right atrium and ventricle (see Box 6.1). The EP protocol for VAs involves paced "PVCs" from various locations in the right ventricle and timed during the T wave in an attempt to provoke (or "induce") VT. If a single-paced PVC fails to induce VT, paced pairs or even triplets are tried. Patients with *ischemic heart disease* who have inducible, sustained VT are at risk

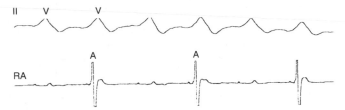

FIGURE 6.8. Wide QRS tachycardia; simultaneous recording of ECG lead II and th right atrial (RA) electrogram. There is not an atrial (A) beat with each ventricular complex (V). AV dissociation indicates VT.

for VF and sudden death. Conversely, when VT cannot be induced in the EP laboratory, the risk of sudden death is relatively low, and implantable cardioverter-defibrillator (ICD) therapy is not indicated.

Unfortunately, provocative EP testing is not as predictive for VF and sudden death for patients with *nonischemic* cardiomyopathy. A negative study does not reliably place the patient in a low risk category. Thus, some experts advocate ICD treatment of symptomatic VT without EP testing.

The EP study may also be used with "wide QRS complex tachycardia" to differentiate VT from SVT with aberrant conduction. The key is to identify the relationship of P waves and QRS complexes (Fig. 6.8). With SVT there is a P wave with each QRS complex. With VT, the atria and ventricles are functioning separately, with "AV dissociation." In rare cases, P waves can be seen on the surface ECG, and EPS is unnecessary, but P waves are usually buried in the QRS complexes. In the EP laboratory an electrode against the atrial wall magnifies P waves.

Treatment of VAs: the Implantable Cardioverter-Defibrillator (ICD)

As noted, we no longer try to suppress PVCs or even nonsustained VT with drug therapy. The routine use of beta-blocker therapy after MI has been shown to lower the risk of sudden death and thus may be considered prophylactic. It may be similarly effective for others with nonischemic cardiomyopathy, as beta blockade has been found to improve survival (see Chapter 1).

TABLE 6.5. Safety of Antiarrhythmic Drug Therapy

Drug Class	Risk
IA Quinidine Procainamide Disopyramide Moricizine	Proarrhythmia* risk is 1–3% if treating isolated PVCs or supraventricular arrhythmias, but 10–15% when treating VT. Torsade is a common arrhythmia and may occur early after starting therapy (monitor the QT interval).
IB Lidocaine Mexiletine Tocainide	Proarrhythmia in 2% when treating PVCs, 5% when treating VT.
IC Flecainide Propafenone	Proarrhythmia in 1% when treating supraventricular arrhythmias and LVEF is normal. With depressed LVEF proarrhythmia is 10–15% (a relative contraindication to these drugs). Look for QRS prolongation. QT prolongation and torsade are uncommon.
III Amiodarone Sotalol	*Amiodarone:* Proarrhythmia in about 1% when the LV is normal, and it goes to only 2% with low LVEF. For this reason, it is our first choice for patients with depressed LV function. *Sotalol:* Proarrhythmia in 2% with normal LVEF and increases to 6–10% with low LVEF. Proarrhythmia is dose dependent with this drug.

*Proarrhythmia is defined as drug-induced VT.

Symptomatic or sustained (≥30 seconds) VT is an indication for EP study for patients with coronary artery disease and probably for nonischemic conditions as well. Inducible sustained VT is the indication for the ICD. The ICD is the most effective therapy for preventing sudden death, with 95% survival at 5 years. It works by first identifying a rapid heart rate. Modern devices often incorporate a pacing protocol to overdrive pace the ventricle and interrupt the VT circuit. If this does not work, the ICD fires, delivering between 15 and 25 J to the endocardial surface. It records the rhythm before firing, documenting the rhythm leading to discharge. The longevity of the battery is determined by the number of discharges, and with "average use" they tend to last 4 to 8 years before a battery change is needed.

Many patients with an ICD also are on VT-suppressing drug therapy (Table 6.5). Although drug therapy may not improve survival when used alone, preventing VT at least prolongs battery life and avoids the discomfort of the device firing.

When the ICD fires, patients are usually admitted for telemetry, especially if symptomatic. Repetitive inappropriate firing can be stopped with a magnet placed over the battery pack. Electrolytes

TABLE 6.6. Illnesses Complicated by VT or Sudden Cardiac Death (SCD)

Illness	Comment
Acute MI	VT or VF are most common during the first 6–12 hours of MI, and may occur with small as well as large infarction (see Chapter 4).
Chronic CAD	Except for the acute phase of MI, the risk VT is highest in those with low LVEF. VT is rare with normal LVEF. *Monomorphic VT* is the usual form of VT with ischemic cardiomyopathy. EPS is a reliable guide to prognosis and treatment.
Dilated nonischemic cardiomyopathy	*Polymorphic VT* is common with dilated cardiomyopathy. EPS is not as predictive, as patients who do not have inducible VT may still have SCD.
Long QT syndrome	Usually acquired (see Table 5.7). Familial long QT may be accompanied by deafness, and this combination carries a high risk for torsade de pointes and SCD. Treat with beta-blockers to keep the peak exercise heart rate < 130 beats/min and possibly with sympthectomy.
Hypertrophic cardiomyopathy (IHSS)	Risk of SCD is increased with a family history of sudden death and history of syncope. SCD is *not* predicted by symptoms, outflow tract gradient, or ECG abnormalities. In fact, SCD may be the initial symptom of hypertrophic cardiomyopathy.
Right ventricular dysplasia	Rare. The ECG shows LBBB, and the VT has a LBBB pattern. Diagnosis is made by echo, and therapy is guided by EPS.
Normal heart VT	Screening for LV dysfunction and CAD are negative. Risk of SCD is low. Radiofrequency ablation is possible.

LBBB, left bundle branch block; CAD, coronary artery disease.

are checked, and a chest x-ray is done to evaluate lead position. A decision for outpatient evaluation is best left to the EP specialist.

Other conditions that may cause VT and sudden cardiac death are reviewed in Table 6.6.

Torsade de Pointes, QT Interval Prolongation, and Proarrhythmia

This is a peculiar form of VT, with wide polymorphic QRS complexes that become larger and then smaller as the axis shifts (Fig. 6.9). It is like the axis is "turning about a point," hence the ballet term, torsade de pointes. It is a "triggered" arrhythmia (not reentrant) that usually occurs when there is a long QT interval (Table 6.7). I first encountered it in the early 1970s in a patient with AF who developed "quinidine syncope," a complication of quinidine

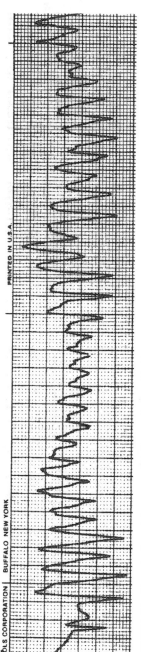

FIGURE 6.9. Torsade de pointes, an undulating, polymorphic VT in which the axis of each successive beat is different from that of the preceding one. (Reproduced by permission from Taylor GJ. 150 Practice ECGs. Cambridge, MA: Blackwell Science, 1997.)

TABLE 6.7. Prolonged QT Interval*

Familial
  Jervell and Lange-Nielsen syndrome (congenital deafness, autosomal recessive)
  Romano-Ward syndrome (normal hearing, autosomal dominant)

Acquired*
  Drugs
    Quinidine
    Procainamide and metabolites
    Sotalol
    Amiodarone
    Disopyramide
    Phenothiazines and derivatives (including some antihistamines)
    Tricyclic antidepressants
    Erythromycin (especially in combination with antihistamines)
    Pentamidine
    Some antimalarial agents
    Cisapride (Propulsid)

  Electrolyte abnormalities
    Hypokalemia and hypomagnesemia (both common with diuretic therapy
      but may also complicate starvation or extreme diets)
    Hypocalcemia (in this case the T wave arrives late, but the T wave is not
      broad; the arrhythmia risk is lower than with other long QT syndromes)

  Others
    Acute myocardial ischemia
    Central nervous system lesions
    Hypothermia
    Bradycardia

---

*The normal QT interval varies with heart, and Bazett's formula corrects for this:
QTc = QT ÷ square root of the RR interval. For the average adult, top normal
QTc < 0.45 seconds.

The conditions and drugs that prolong the QT are synergistic. Thus, a patient on
quinidine who has a drop in magnesium may develop QT prolongation and torsade.

---

therapy subsequently identified as VT. Another patient I treated in the coronary care unit with intractable VT had been on chronic tricyclic antidepressant therapy and had her first episode of syncope the day after starting antihistamines.

Torsade is thus a common form of proarrhythmia and tends to develop early after starting a new drug. Think of it as an idiosyncratic rather than a dose-dependent reaction. Lability of the QT interval is a predictor of sudden cardiac death in patients with long QT. Recent studies have looked at the "QTD," the difference between the longest and shortest QT intervals with ambulatory monitoring. Pause-dependent lengthening of the QT may initiate torsade.

Treatment

Torsade may be prevented by avoiding electrolyte abnormalities or combinations of drugs that prolong the QT (Table 6.7). This is especially important for a patient whose baseline QT interval is long.

The acute arrhythmia is treated using measures that shorten the QT interval. Intravenous magnesium often works. Increasing the heart rate with pacemaker or isoproterenol therapy also shortens the QT and prevents pauses and pause-dependent QT prolongation. Other antiarrhythmic drugs are usually avoided. Hemodynamically unstable VT is treated with DC cardioversion.

Proarrhythmia Without QT Prolongation

The class IC antiarrhythmic drugs (flecainide and propafenone, Table 6.5) delay intraventricular conduction and widen the QRS complex but have less effect on repolarization (the QT interval). The mechanism of proarrhythmia is reentry, and it is dose dependent. To avoid this complication, repeat the ECG a couple weeks after starting the medicine to be sure that the QRS duration has not changed. QRS prolongation may only be present during exercise, and exercise testing may be considered if a patient on IC agents is having "spells." Unlike torsade, which often happens soon after starting the medicine, this drug-induced monomorphic VT may occur late (as in the CAST study, see Table 5.11). VT is more common when LV function is depressed, and use of IC agents should be limited to those with normal LVEF (usually for prevention of AF).

BRADYARRHYTHMIAS

Heart Block

Block can be a confusing term in cardiovascular medicine. Blocked arteries, blocked valves, and blocked nerve conduction are different illnesses. The term *heart block* usually refers to interruption of nerve conduction.

Nerve conduction may be blocked at any level of the cardiac nervous system. It is possible but uncommon within the sinoatrial (SA) node or in the body of the atrium, and is more common in the AV node and the nerves below it. These infranodal nerves include the His-Purkinje system.

Blocked conduction may alter intervals on the ECG and cause bradycardia and syncope. When block is complete, there is no transmission to distal structures, but the heart rarely stops.

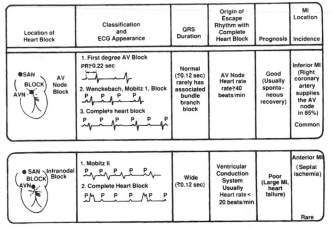

Location of Heart Block		Classification and ECG Appearance	QRS Duration	Origin of Escape Rhythm with Complete Heart Block	Prognosis	MI Location Incidence
•SAN (BLOCK) AVN	AV Node Block	1. First degree AV Block PR≥0.22 sec 2. Wenckebach, Mobitz 1, Block P P P P 3. Complete heart block P P P P P P	Normal (≤0.12 sec) rarely has associated bundle branch block	AV Node Heart rate rate≥40 beats/min	Good (Usually spontaneous recovery)	Inferior MI (Right coronary artery supplies the AV node in 85%) Common
• SAN (BLOCK) AVN	Intranodal Block	1. Mobitz II P P P P P 2. Complete Heart Block P P P P P P P	Wide (≥0.12 sec)	Ventricular Conduction System Usually Heart rate < 20 beats/min	Poor (Large MI, heart failure)	Anterior MI (Septal ischemia) Rare

FIGURE 6.10. Heart block after MI. It is important to distinguish between block at the level of the AV node and block below the AV node. The takeover pacemaker with AV nodal block has an adequate intrinsic rate and responds to atropine. Deep ventricular pacemakers that take over after infranodal block are less responsive and are too slow. (Reproduced by permission from Taylor GJ. 150 Practice ECGs. Cambridge, MA: Blackwell Science, 1997.)

Instead, an auxiliary pacemaker below the level of block takes over. The intrinsic rate of the takeover pacemaker is progressively slower the farther it is from the SA node. Control of heart rate reminds me of the children's game, King of the Mountain. Pacers highest on the mountain, nearest the SA node, get the first chance to rule. When they fail (or their output is blocked), those just below take over. As you go lower on the mountain, the pacers are slower.

For example, when complete block occurs in the AV node, a pacemaker in the His bundle, just below the AV node, takes over with an intrinsic rate of 35 to 45 beats/min (Fig. 6.10). It would be hard to exercise with a heart rate that slow, but with that rate syncope is uncommon. If complete block occurs farther down, within the interventricular septum and beyond the division of the two bundle branches, the takeover pacer is in the body of the ventricles. These deeper pacers have a much slower intrinsic rate, occasionally as slow as 10 to 20 beats/min. In this case, syncope and even sudden death are possible.

In addition to a slower intrinsic rate, takeover pacers in the ventricle are less responsive to the autonomic nervous system. A pacemaker in the AV node, or just below it, may still respond to catecholamine stimulation with an increase in the rate of firing.

From this outline of general principles, you begin to see that the level of block determines prognosis, and identification of this level is critical.

First-degree AV Block

First-degree heart block is defined as a PR interval at least 0.22 seconds. The level of conduction delay is the AV node. Increased vagal tone, hyperkalemia, digitalis, calcium channel blockers (diltiazem and verapamil), and β-adrenergic blockers all may slow AV conduction. It is common in elderly people who may have primary degeneration of the AV node in the absence of ischemic heart disease. In others, ischemia may injure the AV node and delay or block conduction. The right coronary artery usually supplies the AV node and the inferior wall of the heart. AV nodal block is thus common with inferior MI (Fig. 6.10).

Second-degree Heart Block

Mobitz I (Wenckebach) and II Block With second-degree AV block, some beats pass through the AV node to the ventricles, but others do not. It usually follows a pattern; when every other P wave captures the ventricle (producing a QRS complex), the patient is said to have 2 to 1 (2:1) block. When every third P wave is conducted through the AV node, it is 3:1 block, and when two of three P waves are conducted, it is 3:2 block.

Second-degree block is further classified into two types, *Mobitz I and II*. I find this confusing. It is easier to remember without the Mobitz designations, instead thinking anatomically of where in the conduction block occurs.

Mobitz I block usually occurs within the AV node (exceptions are rare). The dysfunctional node tires with each succeeding beat until it is so tired that a P wave is completely blocked. On the ECG, there is progressive prolongation of the PR interval until a P wave is blocked and not followed by a QRS (Fig. 6.11). This is also called the Wenckebach phenomenon. Notice that the

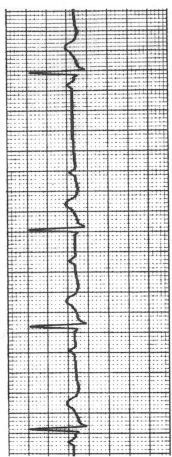

FIGURE 6.11. Second-degree AV block, Mobitz type I (or Wenckebach). The level of block is the AV node. There is progressive lengthening of the PR interval until the P wave is not conducted. After the dropped beat, the PR interval is short (the AV node has had time to recuperate). An additional feature, not mentioned in the text, is progressive shortening of the RR interval before the dropped beat. Note that the QRS complex is narrow, more evidence that the level of block is the AV node. (Reproduced by permission from Taylor GJ. 150 Practice ECGs. Cambridge, MA: Blackwell Science, 1997.)

PR interval after the totally blocked P wave is short, reflecting recuperation of the node.

The conduction system below the AV node is usually normal in patients with Mobitz I block. With normal intraventricular conduction, the right and left ventricles are activated simultaneously and the QRS duration is normal. A narrow QRS excludes block below the AV node. On the other hand, a wide QRS does not guarantee that block is infranodal, because a patient with pre-existing infranodal disease (and bundle branch block) may develop AV nodal block.

Mobtiz II block is caused by block below the AV node. It does not cause progressive prolongation of the PR in the beats before the blocked P wave (Fig. 6.12). Because the infranodal conduction system is diseased, the QRS is wide. A narrow QRS excludes infranodal heart block. Mobitz II block often precedes symptomatic complete heart block and is an indicator for pacemaker implantation for a patient with syncope or near-syncope.

2:1 Block: Is It Mobitz I or II? Mobitz I second-degree AV block can be severe enough that every other beat is blocked. This would eliminate progressive lengthening of the PR interval as a diagnostic marker of AV nodal rather than infranodal block. It is a common occurrence with digitalis toxicity.

There are a couple of ways to tell the level of block. One is to get a long rhythm strip, looking for times where block is less severe, with 3:2 or 4:3 conduction and typical PR interval findings. Another is to focus on the QRS duration. If narrow, the block is nodal. If wide, it may be infranodal (check an old ECG; a narrow QRS previously but a wide one now suggests new infranodal conduction disease).

The final and most accurate method for determining the level of AV block is a His bundle recording in the EP laboratory (Fig. 6.13). A long H-V interval indicating infranodal conduction disease would favor pacemaker therapy.

Third-degree Complete Heart Block
Nothing gets through. There are P waves and QRS complexes, but they are unrelated (Fig. 6.14). This is an example of *AV dissociation* (another is VT with an unrelated atrial rhythm, Fig. 6.8). How do you know whether complete block is at the level of the AV node or below it?

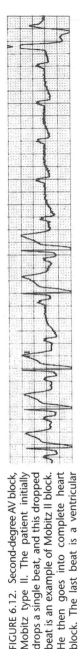

FIGURE 6.12. Second-degree AV block, Mobitz type II. The patient initially drops a single beat, and this dropped beat is an example of Mobitz II block. He then goes into complete heart block. The last beat is a ventricular escape beat. The PR interval of conducted beats is fixed; there is no evidence of the Wenckebach phenomenon. In addition, the QRS complex is wide; the 12-lead ECG showed bifascicular block (see Chapter 2). A wide QRS, indicating abnormal intraventricular conduction, is invariable seen in patients with infranodal heart block. (Reproduced by permission from Taylor GJ. 150 Practice ECGs. Cambridge, MA: Blackwell Science, 1997.)

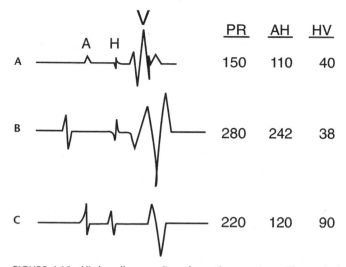

	PR	AH	HV
A	150	110	40
B	280	242	38
C	220	120	90

FIGURE 6.13. His bundle recordings from three patients. The goal of EPS when evaluating heart block is to determine the anatomic level of conduction delay (see Fig. 6.11). The His (H) spike is generated by depolarization of the His bundle, just below and adjacent to the AV node, and is recorded with a bipolar catheter positioned next to the tricuspid valve. The H spike essentially divides the PR interval into its AV nodal (the AH interval) and infranodal (HV) portions. Patient A: the PR interval is normal as is the HV interval (<55 msec). Patient B: A patient with first-degree AV block (long PR). Marked prolongation of the AH interval indicates that the level of block is the AV node. Infranodal conduction (the HV interval) is normal. Patient C: Another with first-degree AV block. The AH interval is normal, so there is no delay in conduction in the AV node. The prolonged HV interval indicates infranodal conduction delay. With infranodal disease there is a higher risk of developing symptomatic heart block. (Reproduced by permission from Taylor GJ. Primary care management of heart disease. St. Louis, MO: Mosby, 2000.)

The issues are those discussed above with 2:1 AV block. When block is at the level of the node, the QRS is usually narrow, the takeover pacing rate is above 40 beats/min, and the rate increases with isoproterenol or atropine therapy. This is the usual case with congenital complete heart block.

Infranodal complete heart block is more common with elderly patients. It usually causes syncope (Stokes-Adams attacks) but may present as fatigue or heart failure. Even if it is asymptomatic it is an indication for permanent pacing, because sudden death is possible. The etiology is often misunderstood. Senile

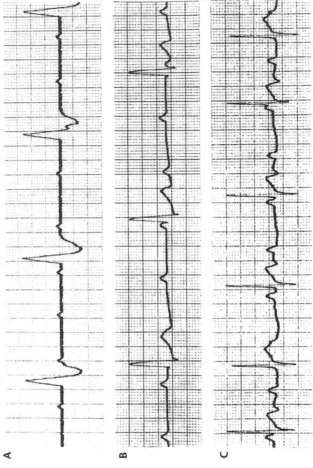

FIGURE 6.14. Three patients with complete heart block. The atria are being discharged at a regular rate (P waves) and the ventricles at a regular rate (QRS complexes). The two rhythms appear unrelated; there is *AV dissociation*. You may be tempted to say that P waves coming before QRS could be conducted, but these do not alter the regularity of the ventricular escape rhythm. Patients A and B have wide QRS complexes and slow ventricular rates; they probably have block below the AV node, and the takeover pacemakers are ventricular in origin. Patient C has a more rapid escape rate (55 beats/min), and the QRS complex is narrow; the level of block is probably the AV node. (Reproduced by permission from Taylor GJ. 150 Practice ECGs. Cambridge, MA: Blackwell Science, 1997.)

A

B

C

244

heart block is *not* caused by coronary artery disease. Instead, a degenerative fibrotic process involving cardiac nerves below the AV node is the usual cause. One of my teachers referred to "frayed wires." Most of these patients have bundle branch block preceding their third-degree block. Unless there are other symptoms indicating ischemia, evaluation for coronary artery disease is unnecessary.

Sick Sinus Syndrome

Sick sinus syndrome, also called the brady-tachy syndrome, usually occurs in elderly patients and is the most common indication for pacemaker therapy in the United States. It is defined as abnormal sinus node function that correlates with symptoms. Patients often have atrial tachyarrhythmias (including PSVT and AF) and spells of marked sinus bradycardia. Bouts of tachycardia may be followed by disturbingly long SA pauses with syncope. EPS is rarely needed to make the diagnosis. When done, testing sinus node function in the EP laboratory involves rapid atrial pacing and determining how long it takes the SA node to fire when pacing is terminated (the "sinus node recovery time").

Drug therapy that is needed to control the fast rhythm usually aggravates the bradyarrhythmia. A combination of drug and pacemaker treatment is often required.

Pacemaker Therapy

The most common indication for cardiac pacing is a symptomatic bradyarrhythmia. It is important to document the slow rhythm while the patient is symptomatic. Prophylactic pacing is justified for complete heart block, asystolic pauses at least 4 seconds in duration, and after anterior MI when there is new left bundle branch block or bifascicular block. As noted in Chapter 5, permanent pacing is seldom needed after inferior MI and third-degree heart block, because spontaneous recovery is the rule.

Pacemaker Nomenclature

A three-letter code is used to describe pacemakers. The first letter refers to the chamber that is paced, the second to the chamber sensed, and the third to the "mode of response" (inhibited or triggered). Single-chamber VVI pacing is still commonly used: a lead in the right ventricle paces the heart and the same ventricular lead is the sensor. If the heart rate is adequate, the pacer senses this and "inhibits" itself for a preset period of time. If it senses no ventricular beat (there is a pause), it paces the ventricle.

For some time, dual-chamber pacemakers had a pacing electrode in the right ventricle and only a sensing electrode in the right atrium. This sensed P waves and "triggered" a ventricular beat (VAT pacing).

Modern dual-chamber pacers are DDD; they pace both the atrium and ventricle and sense in both places. When the atrial lead senses P waves, it inhibits atrial pacing. And if the ventricular lead does not sense a QRS on time, it triggers ventricular pacing.

Physiology of Pacing

Single-chamber ventricular pacing protects against slow heart rate. However, it bypasses atrial contraction, and the atrial contribution to diastolic filling is lost. Normally, this lowers cardiac output by 10% to 15% (see Fig. 1.8). This may be intolerable for the patient with heart failure and borderline compensation. Others with diastolic dysfunction are even more "preload dependent." Because of poor LV diastolic compliance, loss of atrial contraction may lower cardiac output by 25% or more. Elderly patients often have increased ventricular stiffness, and they are the ones who usually need pacemakers.

A clinical consequence of VVI pacing may be the "pacemaker syndrome." The patient describes spells of fatigue or weakness—caused by an abrupt fall in cardiac output—whenever the ventricular pacemaker turns on. The solution is dual-chamber pacing, which preserves atrial contraction.

DDD pacing is thus useful when there is abnormal systolic or diastolic LV function. Note that DDD pacing is not possible when the underlying rhythm is AF.

Temporary Transcutaneous Pacing

This temporary pacemaker device is the method of choice for stabilizing patients with an acute bradyarrhythmia. Blind placement of a transvenous pacing electrode in an acute setting rarely works, even when the operator is experienced.

Large pads are placed on the anterior and posterior chest, and electricity passing between the electrodes stimulates the heart. One area of potential confusion is that the pacing spikes are huge, and nurses must reduce the gain on the telemetry ECG.

The QRS complex essentially disappears, and it may seem that the pacemaker is not capturing. If the patient has a pulse, the pacemaker is working.

Pacemaker Follow-up and Troubleshooting

All patients are enrolled in a pacemaker telephone follow-up clinic. Regular telephone monitoring using a fingertip electrode and a transmitter allows troubleshooting. Pacemaker leads and batteries may fail unexpectedly, and failure is easily detected with telephone telemetry. A drop in the baseline pacing rate indicates that the battery is reaching end-of-life.

If the pacemaker is not firing at all in the patient with a normal heart rate, the patient places a magnet over the battery. This temporarily turns the sensing function off, and the pacer fires at its fixed rate (ensuring us that the pacer still works). You may use a magnet in a similar fashion in the emergency room to establish fixed rate pacing (DOO or VOO pacing).

Electrical Interference Pacemaker shielding is effective. Household appliances, microwave ovens, and cellular telephones are not a problem, although I recommend not having the pacemaker battery in direct contact with the device. Powerful electromagnetic sources such as a ham radio or an arc welder may be more dangerous, and the pacemaker company should be consulted before their use. Elective DC cardioversion is safe, with the electrodes positioned anterior-posterior, away from the pacemaker battery. In like fashion, electroconvulsive therapy, electrocautery during surgery, and lithotripsy are safe as long as they do not direct energy to the region of the pacemaker battery.

On the other hand, magnetic resonance imaging subjects the pacemaker to intense magnetic fields and is generally contraindicated. Radiation therapy may alter pacer function if the battery is directly in the radiation beam. In both cases, if absolutely needed consult the pacemaker company.

SYNCOPE

The sudden loss of consciousness with reduced cerebral blood flow usually occurs when systolic blood pressure falls below 70 mm Hg. A fall in cardiac output is the cause in most cases, and common etiologies are reviewed in Table 6.8.

TABLE 6.8. Syncope

Cardiac Causes	Comment
Slow heart rate causing low cardiac output	Heart block (Stokes-Adams attacks), asystole, atrial fibrillation with slow ventricular rate (common in elderly patients with AV node degeneration). All may be aggravated by digitalis, beta-blocker, verapamil, and diltiazem.
Rapid ventricular rhythms	Review Tables 5.6 and 5.7.
Mechanical causes of low cardiac output	*Left heart:* aortic stenosis, hypertrophic cardiomyopathy and LV outflow obstruction, atrial myxoma, prosthetic valve malfunction. Rarely syncope complicates mitral stenosis and aortic regurgitation. *Right heart:* pulmonary embolism, primary pulmonary hypertension, pulmonic stenosis, Eisenmenger's syndrome, tetralogy of Fallot (pulmonary outflow obstruction); pericardial tamponade (reduce cardiac filling).
Pacemaker failure	Loss of pacing and severe bradycardia, pacer-induced tachyarrhythmia, the "pacemaker syndrome" (an abrupt drop in cardiac output when the ventricular pacer turns on and there is loss of atrial contraction, see text).
Neurocardiogenic syncope	See text

table continues

A patient's other cardiac or medical history may point to an etiology. Thus, a history of prior MI or heart failure suggests VT as the cause. An elderly person with no prior cardiac history may have intermittent complete heart block, especially if the ECG shows bundle branch block. The treatment of cardiac arrhythmias causing syncope has been reviewed. Arrhythmias are uncommon in otherwise healthy younger patients; think instead of neurocardiogenic or carotid sinus syncope, and screen for other cardiac lesions that may not be apparent on physical exam (Table 6.8).

Neurocardiogenic Syncope

Before the discovery of this illness, about one half the patients with syncope were labeled idiopathic. Neurocardiogenic syncope, often called vasovagal syncope and a variant orthostatic hypotension, is responsible for most of these cases.

The Reflex

The initiating event is venous pooling with a shift to upright posture. Reduced venous return leads to lower cardiac output.

TABLE 6.8. *(continued)*

Noncardiac causes	Comment
Vasovagal syncope	The common faint, and the mechanism is similar to that of neurocardiogenic syncope. Always a prodrome: sweats, pallor, nausea, blurred vision. This differentiates it from the "drop attack" that occurs with cardiac arrhythmias.
Orthostatic hypotension	Often associated with antihypertensive drug therapy and also with phenothiazines, antidepressants, and tranquilizers.
Cerebrovascular disease	Vertebrobasilar insufficiency is a rare (about 6%) complication of TIA or stroke, and other brainstem symptoms are the rule (vertigo, diplopia, dysarthria, paresthesia, ataxia).
Subclavian steal syndrome	Follows upper extremity exertion. Look for a pulse deficit on the stenosed side and a bruit. Mechanism: occlusion of the subclavian artery. With arm exertion and vasodilatation, flow is "stolen" from the vertebral artery, the source of collateral flow to the stenosed vessel. Brainstem ischemia causes syncope.
Carotid sinus syncope	Usually elderly patients. About 25% report symptoms with stimulation of the carotid sinus (sudden turns, shaving, a tight collar). Others have hypertension or CAD. A few have pathologic conditions of the neck (tumor, prior radiation, large lymph nodes, prior trauma).
Situational syncope	Micturition, cough or sneeze, defecation and straining, swallowing and Valsalva syncope. Vagal activation is the usual mechanism
Migraine syndromes	Syncope is possible, but other features of migraine are usually present.
Metabolic	Hypoglycemia, hypoxia, hyperventilation.
Hysterical syncope	

TIA, transient ischemic attack; CAD, coronary artery disease.

Baroreceptors are stimulated, increasing adrenergic tone. Both heart rate and contractility increase. This is the normal response to upright posture and decreased venous return.

For uncertain reasons, patients with neurally mediated syncope have an overshoot of the reaction of LV mechanoreceptors to this increase in contractility (receptors that also are responsible for the Bezold-Jarish reflex). These receptors are connected to the central vasomotor center, and there are two responses to vasomotor center activation: *vagal discharge*, leading to decreased heart rate and, rarely, asystole, and *withdrawal of sympathetic tone*, leading to vasodilation and hypotension. In most cases hypotension is the predominant mechanism leading to syncope (Fig. 6.15).

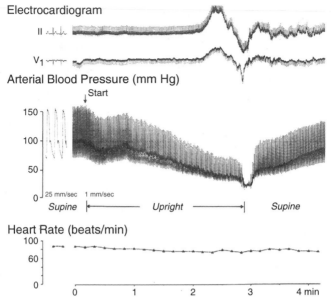

FIGURE 6.15. Tilt-table test in a 72-year-old woman with breast cancer metastatic to the glossopharyngeal region. This episode of syncope occurred despite a dual-chamber pacemaker and stable heart rate. Note that pressure fell slowly but steadily with head-up tilt, and syncope occurred 3 minutes later. She was successfully treated with disopyramide. (Reproduced by permission from Oswald S, Trouton T. Neurocardiogenic (vasodepressed) syncope. N Engl J Med 1993;329:30.)

Clinical Features and Evaluation

Of note, this complex series of reflexes takes some time. The patient is usually upright for 2 to 5 minutes before dizziness begins. A typical history is "I got up, walked to the kitchen, and fell while standing at the sink." Syncope may occur while sitting and with standing.

You may try to elicit symptoms at the bedside, having the patient stand and monitoring blood pressure for 5 to 10 minutes. More sensitive is the *tilt-table test,* which monitors arterial pressure even longer. One study reported a mean time to syncope of 12 minutes. Strapping the patient to the tilt table avoids muscular activity that may prevent the initial vagal response. The sensitivity of this test may be increased by repeating it with isoproterenol infusion, although this reduces specificity (more false positives).

Treatment

The treatment goals are augmentation of vascular volume and blocking the inappropriate increase in LV contractility. Low-dose beta blockade works for most patients. Diuretics should be stopped if possible, and salt tablets may be added. Disopyramide (which reduces contractility); clonidine (which inhibits the central vasomotor center); scopolamine (a vagolytic); fludrocortisone (which promotes salt retention); or ephedrine, phenylephrine, or midroine (vasoconstrictors) may also be used.

SUGGESTED READINGS _____

Atrial Arrhythmias

A-Khatib SM, Pritchett EL. Clinical features of Wolff-Parkinson-White syndrome. Am Heart J 1999;138:403–413. (The first of a comprehensive three-part review.)

DiMarco JP, Miles W, Akhtar M, et al. Adenosine for paroxysmal SVT. Ann Intern Med 1990;113:104–110.

Fenelon G, Wijns W, Andries E, Burgada P. Tachycardiomyopathy: mechanisms and clinical implications. Pacing Clin Electrophysiol 1996;19:95–103.

Hart RG, Halperin JL. Atrial fibrillation and thromboembolism: a decade of progress in stroke prevention. Ann Intern Med 1999;131:768–795. (There is a sixfold increase in stroke risk, and warfarin reduces this by 60%. Good review of the randomized trials and patient selection issues [who needs warfarin vs. aspirin].)

Hewitt RL, Chun KL, Flint LM. Current clinical concepts in perioperative anticoagulation. Am Surg 1999;65:270–273. (Patients with nonvalvular AF or prosthetic valves are not at sufficient risk of arterial embolism to justify full dose heparin therapy during the brief perioperative period. If there has been a recent thromboembolic event, heparin is needed.)

Jagasia DH, Williams B, Ezekowitz MD. Clinical implication of antiembolic trials in atrial fibrillation and role of transesophageal echocardiography in atrial fibrillation. Curr Opin Cardiol 2000; 15:58–63. (Identifies the cutoff age for warfarin therapy as 75 years.)

Manolis AS, Wang PJ, Estes NA. Radiofrequency catheter ablation for cardiac tachyarrhythmias. Ann Intern Med 1994;121: 452–461.

Oral H, Souza JJ, Michaud GF, et al. Facilitating transthoracic cardioversion of atrial fibrillation with ibutilide pretreatment. N Engl J Med 1999;340:1849–1854.

Seidl K, Hauer B, Schwick NG, et al. Risk of thromboembolic events in patients with atrial flutter. Am J Cardiol 1998;82: 580–586. (Documented embolism in 11 of 191 consecutive patients with chronic atrial flutter. The risk of embolism is less than it is with atrial fibrillation, and there are no clinical trial data to guide treatment of atrial flutter. However, I now apply the AF anticoagulation guidelines in cases of atrial flutter.)

Stevenson WG, Stevenson LW. Atrial fibrillation in heart failure. N Engl J Med 1999;341:910–911. (Only amiodarone has been sufficiently studied to determine that it does not increase the risk of death among patients with heart failure.)

Tomita M, Ikeguchi S, Kagawa K, et al. Serial histopathologic myocardial findings in a patient with ectopic atrial tachycardia-induced cardiomyopathy. J Cardiol 1997;29:37–42. (Despite normalization of LVEF with correction of the tachycardia, myocardial fibrosis persisted suggesting permanent damage. A common issue is how long to continue afterload reduction therapy. It may be sensible to continue it for a year [or longer], as the heart may not have recovered completely just because LVEF has normalized. The same argument could be made with other causes of cardiomyopathy that have appeared to improve.)

Ventricular Arrhythmias

Cardiac Arrhythmia Suppression Trial (CAST) Investigators. Preliminary report: effect of encainide and flecainide on mortality in a randomized trial of arrhythmia suppression after myocardial infarction. N Engl J Med 1989;321:406–413. (A landmark study, one that you should be able to cite after your cardiology rotation.)

Friedman PL, Stevenson WG. Proarrhythmia. Am J Cardiol 1998;82:50N–58N.

Fu EY, Clemo HF, Ellenbogen KA. Acquired QT prolongation: mechanism and implications. Cardiol Rev 1998;6:319–326. (A thorough review of torsade de pointes.)

Greene HL. The implantable cardioverter-defibrillator. Clin Cardiol 2000;23:315–326. (A thorough review, including advice on management of the patient who has experienced a shock. Note that troponin may be raised by multiple shocks.)

Janeira LF. Wide-complex tachycardias. The importance of identifying the mechanism. Postgrad Med 1996;100:259–272. (A review of ECG criteria for differentiating PVCs from aberrantly conducted atrial ectopics.)

Kennedy HL, Whitlock JA, Sprague MK, et al. Long-term follow-up of asymptomatic healthy subjects with frequent and complex ventricular ectopy. N Engl J Med 1985;312:193–199.

Kowey PR, Marinchak RA, Rials SF, et al. Intravenous antiarrhythmic therapy in the acute control of in-hospital destabilizing
ventricular tachycardia and fibrillation. Am J Cardiol 1999;84:46–51.

Link MS, Wang PL, Maron BJ, Estes NAM. What is *commotio
cordis*? Cardiol Rev 1999;7:265–269. (A newly described cause of
ventricular tachycardia and sudden death. Blunt nonpenetrating
chest wall trauma [e.g., a blow from a baseball or hockey puck] provokes a PVC that triggers VT or VF and sudden death. The blow
may seem innocuous. One cause of sudden death in young athletes.)

Multicenter Automatic Defibrillator Implantation Trial Investigators. Improve survival with an implanted defibrillator in patients
with coronary disease at high risk for ventricular arrhythmia. N
Engl J Med 1996;335:1933–1940.

Naccarella R, Lepera G, Rolli A. Arrhythmic risk stratification
of post-myocardial infarction patients. Curr Opin Cardiol 2000;
15:1–6.

Naccarelli GV, Wolbrette DL, Del'Orfano JT, et al. Amiodarone: what have we learned from clinical trials. Clin Cardiol
2000;23:73–82.

Roden DM. A practical approach to torsade de pointes. Clin
Cardiol 1997;20:285–292.

Watkins J. Sudden death in hypertrophic cardiomyopathy. N
Engl J Med 2000:342:422–424.

Zimetbaum P, Josephson ME. Evaluation of patients with palpitations. N Engl J Med 1998;338:1369–1374.

Bradyarrhythmias, Pacing, and Syncope

Bass EB, Elson JJ, Fogoros RN, et al. Long-term prognosis of
patients undergoing electrophysiologic studies for syncope of unknown
origin. Am J Cardiol 1988;62:1186–1192.

Benditt DG, Fahy GJ, Lurie KG, et al. Pharmacotherapy of
neurally mediated syncope. Circulation 1999;100:1242–1248.

Bloomfield DM, Sheldon R, Grubb BP, et al. Putting it
together: and new treatment algorithm for vasovagal syncope and
related disorders. Am J Cardiol 1999;84:33Q–39Q. (There are multiple solid review articles in this symposium.)

Furman JM, Cass SP. Benign paroxysmal positional vertigo. N
Engl J Med 1999;341:1590–1596.

Grubb BP. Pathophysiology and differential diagnosis of neurocardiogenic syncope. Am J Cardiol 1999;84:3Q–9Q.

Kapoor WN, Hammill SC, Gersh BJ. Diagnosis and natural
history of syncope and the role of invasive electrophysiologic testing.

Am J Cardiol 1989;63:730–739. (Still an excellent review, although much that is known about neurocardiogenic syncope has evolved since this article.)

Ling CA, Crouch MA. Theophylline for chronic symptomatic bradycardia in the elderly. Ann Pharmacother 1998;32:837–839. (Consider this approach when pacing has been refused.)

Maron BJ, Nishimura RA, McKenna WJ, et al. Assessment of permanent dual-chamber pacing as a treatment for drug-refractory symptomatic patients with obstructive hypertrophic cardiomyopathy. Circulation 1999;99:2927–2933. (The first randomized trial to assess this therapy, and it did not seem to help most patients. A few elderly patients benefited.)

McComb JM, Gribbin GM. Effect of pacing mode and morbidity and mortality: update of clinical pacing trials. Am J Cardiol 1999;83:211D–213D. (There have been no randomized trials, but retrospective studies suggest that dual chamber pacing reduces morbidity and mortality.)

Moses HW, Moulton KP, Miller BD, Schneider, JA. A practical guide to cardiac pacing, 5th ed. Boston: Little, Brown, 2000. (An excellent primer on pacemaker therapy and a good choice for your library of medical "basics." It is thorough yet short enough to read in three evenings.)

CHAPTER 7

The Consult Service

This chapter briefly touches on other clinical issues you may encounter on the inpatient consult service or on the board exams. It, and this text, does not presume to be comprehensive, but instead represents my choice of clinical issues to cover for your basic data set. (Drop me a note if you feel there are other subjects that should be mentioned.)

PREOPERATIVE EVALUATION OF THE PATIENT HAVING NONCARDIAC SURGERY

"Clearance" For Surgery

Coronary artery disease (CAD) is ubiquitous, and a major risk of general anesthesia and surgery is myocardial ischemia. Primary care doctors and cardiologists are asked to assess cardiac risk and to "clear the patient for surgery."

Identification of high- or low-risk patients is straightforward because it is evidence based. Prospective studies gathered clinical data before surgery, monitored patients for cardiac complications during and after the operation, and identified risk factors. The findings of multiple studies are in general agreement and form the basis of the risk assessment protocols offered by the American College of Physicians (ACP) and the American College of Cardiology. We use the ACP practice guidelines because they are especially well organized (Fig. 7.1 and Tables 7.1 and 7.2).

Almost all the data used to define the patient's risk come from the history and physical examination. When using this algorithm, there are two screening stages.

- Level 1 screen: The "cardiac risk index" is calculated using clinical features that predict myocardial infarction (MI) or cardiac death after surgery (Table 7.1). High-risk patients,

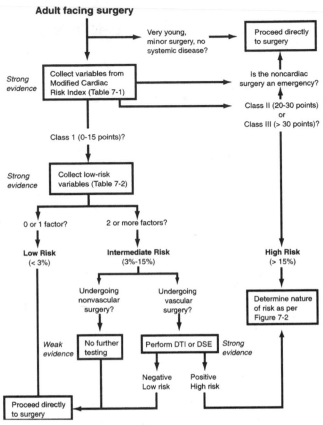

FIGURE 7.1. An algorithm for the assessment of cardiac risk before noncardiac surgery. Boxed phrases indicate recommended actions. Italicized words beside the boxes indicate the level of evidence supporting the recommendation. If no italicized word is present, no evidence exists for or against use. Percentages indicate the chance of a cardiac complication of surgery, usually MI or cardiac death. DTI, dipyridamole thallium imaging; DSE, dobutamine stress echocardiography. (Reproduced by permission from American College of Physicians. Guidelines for assessing and managing the perioperative risk from coronary artery disease associated with major noncardiac surgery. Ann Intern Med 1997;127:309.)

with an index of at least 20 points, have a risk of cardiac complications that exceeds 15%. Figure 7.2 is an algorithm for management of those at high risk. This may involve further study. For example, a patient with recent MI may need

TABLE 7.1. Cardiac Risk Index for Patients Having Noncardiac Surgery*

Variable	Points
Myocardial infarction	
<6 months earlier	10
>6 months earlier	5
Canadian Cardiovascular Society angina class†	
Class III	10
Class IV	20
Alveolar pulmonary edema	
Within the last week	10
Ever	5
Suspected critical aortic stenosis	20
Arrhythmias	
Rhythm other than sinus or sinus plus premature atrial beats	5
>5 premature ventricular contractions on the 12-lead ECG	5
Poor general medical status defined as any of the following:	5
PO_2 < 60 mm Hg, PCO_2 > 50 mm Hg, potassium < 3 mEq/L, creatinine> 2.6, bedridden	
Age > 70 years	5
Emergency surgery	10

*Risk index: class I risk, 0–15 points, class II, 20–30, class III, more than 30 points.
†Canadian Cardiovascular Society classification of angina: class 0, asymptomatic; I, angina with strenuous exercise; II, angina with moderate exertion; III, angina when walking 1 to 2 level blocks or climbing 1 flight of stairs at a normal pace; IV, inability to perform any physical activity without angina.
Source: American College of Physicians. Ann Intern Med 1997;127:309.

TABLE 7.2. Low-Risk Variables

Criterial of Eagle et al.*	Criteria of Vanzetto et al.†
Age > 70 years	Age > 70 years
History of angina	History of angina
Diabetes mellitus	Diabetes mellitus
Q waves on the ECG	Q waves on the ECG
History of ventricular ectopy	History of myocardial infarction
	Ischemic ST segment changes on the resting ECG
	Hypertension plus LV hypertrophy on the ECG
	History of congestive heart failure

These criteria are applied to low risk patients to decide who should have preoperative screening for CAD (see text and Fig. 7.1).
*From American College of Physicians. Ann Intern Med 1997;127:309.
†Vanzetto G, et al. Am J Cardiol 1996;77:143.

either perfusion imaging or angiography to determine the risk of more ischemia during surgery.

- Level 2 screen: After the initial screen, those at low risk (scoring less than 20 points) are screened a second time using "low-risk variables" (Table 7.2). With one or none of these

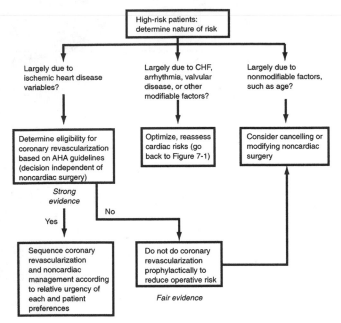

FIGURE 7.2. An algorithm for the management of patients at high risk for perioperative cardiac complications. Boxed phrases indicate recommended actions, and italicized words below the boxes indicate the level of evidence supporting the recommendation. If no italicized word is present, no evidence exists for or against use. AHA, American Heart Association; CHF, congestive heart failure. (Reproduced by permission from American College of Physicians. Guidelines for assessing and managing the perioperative risk from coronary artery disease associated with major noncardiac surgery. Ann Intern Med 1997;127:309.)

risk factors, the chance of a cardiac complication is less than 3%, and the patient goes to surgery without further evaluation (Fig. 7.1). At this low level of risk, stress testing and perfusion imaging do not allow further risk stratification. Note that low risk does not mean zero risk; the patient is always taking a chance when having anesthesia or surgery and should understand that. On the consult, I state that "the risk of surgery and anesthesia is average for the patient's age, and no further cardiac testing is indicated."

Those with two or more of the low-risk variables are in an intermediate risk group and possibly should be screened for CAD with perfusion imaging or stress-echo (Fig. 7.1). This is a large number of patients, as many as half of those you will see as the preoperative medicine consultant. The algorithm indicates that CAD screening is required only for the intermediate-risk patient having vascular surgery. However, it hedges a bit by pointing out that evidence is weak for avoiding screening before nonvascular operations. In the American Heart Association guidelines, exercise tolerance is used to further screen such patients. The intermittent-risk patient who finds it difficult to exercise at the 4 MET level (see Table 4.2), roughly equivalent to walking upstairs to the second floor, and who is having major surgery also deserves noninvasive screening for CAD. But when exercise tolerance is normal, the screening study is not recommended.

Risk of the Operation

More than half of those having vascular surgery also have CAD. Accordingly, the risk of a cardiac event is highest with vascular procedures (a 13% chance of a cardiac complication), just as high with orthopedic surgery, and is followed by abdominal and thoracic (8%), head and neck, ophthalmic, and prostate operations (3%). Emergency surgery, operations lasting more than 5 hours, and procedures that are hemodynamically stressful are higher risk.

Laboratory Testing

Highest and lowest risk patients are readily identified using clinical variables (Table 7.1). It is the intermediate-risk patient who may benefit from noninvasive screening tests (Table 7.2).

The stress electrocardiogram (ECG) is of uncertain usefulness. Many of the illnesses requiring surgery preclude treadmill testing. The ACP guidelines conclude that the stress ECG is not reliable even when a "diagnostic test" is achieved, although the American Heart Association guidelines indicate that it is reliable. In general, most agree that cardiac imaging is a more powerful screening tool, and that is our usual practice.

Pharmacologic stress imaging has the largest and best record of performance, and dipyridamole or adenosine perfusion scanning and dobutamine stress echocardiography are both effective. One study of intermediate-risk patients found a 1% incidence of MI or cardiac death with a negative perfusion scan compared with a 23% risk when the scan showed reversible ischemia. With an imaging study that shows no active ischemia, no further cardiac evaluation is indicated. Note that a person with prior MI may have a fixed perfusion abnormality, a scar, but no reversible ischemia; no further testing is required by this result.

Measurement of left ventricular (LV) ejection fraction is not part of routine screening protocols. It may be helpful in sorting out dyspnea of uncertain cause or to establish a diagnosis of heart failure.

Perioperative Management

The risk of noncardiac surgery is lower after coronary revascularization. However, getting the patient through a noncardiac operation is rarely the only indication for bypass surgery or angioplasty. Instead, the usual indications apply (e.g., unstable coronary syndromes, intolerable symptoms, or high-risk anatomy).

A patient who remains asymptomatic after revascularization requires no special study. Although not supported by clinical trials, some believe that screening for ischemia should be reserved for the asymptomatic patient who had bypass surgery more than 5 to 8 years earlier.

Beta Blockade

The Multicenter Study of Perioperative Ischemia Research found that atenolol given throughout hospitalization lowered the risk of cardiac events by 15% and mortality by 8%. Patient selection criteria for this treatment included known CAD or two risk factors for CAD (in this study, age at least 65 years, current smoking, hypertension, diabetes, or cholesterol at least 240 mg/dL) and no contraindications to beta blockade. Those with heart rates below 55 beats/min were excluded.

The protocol included atenolol 5 mg intravenously 30 minutes before surgery and again just after surgery and then atenolol 50–100 mg orally each day depending on baseline heart rate. Those unable to take oral medications were given 5–10 mg atenolol intravenously at 12-hour intervals.

Other Cardiac Illnesses

Critical aortic stenosis should be repaired before elective noncardiac surgery. Endocarditis prophylaxis is a consideration for all with valvular or congenital disease. In general, antibiotic coverage is indicated for drainage of an infected site or for oral, lower gastrointestinal, gallbladder, and genitourinary procedures (see Chapter 2).

It is important to identify congestive heart failure preoperatively, because it alters the prognosis and changes management. The patient should be at dry weight at the time of surgery. Fluid overload should be avoided after surgery, and careful monitoring of fluid status and electrolytes is needed. Remember that low magnesium and potassium increase the risk of arrhythmias after surgery (see Chapter 6). Magnesium often falls after large operations (the reason is uncertain, but there is speculation that freshly cut tissue soaks up magnesium), and this may be aggravated by diuretic therapy.

RIGHT HEART FAILURE

The most common cause of right heart failure is left heart failure. Yet we encounter an occasional patient with peripheral edema or ascites in the absence of liver disease who has never had pulmonary congestion and who has normal LV ejection fraction and LV diastolic pressure. Let us review a few of the causes of isolated systemic congestion.

Pericardial Disease

Both pericardial tamponade and constriction limit cardiac filling. Consider them "external" causes of right heart failure. The right atrium and ventricle are compressed and just cannot accommodate normal volume. This inadequate preload (as that is what it is) results in reduced stroke volume (see Chapter 1).

Clinically, acute tamponade causes a precipitous fall in blood pressure; a good example is cardiac rupture after MI (see Chapter 5). Chronic pericardial disease presents with symptoms of low cardiac output such as fatigue or weakness and with systemic congestion. I have seen a few cases of "cryptogenic cirrhosis" and massive ascites that turned out to be constrictive pericarditis (one such patient was preparing for liver transplantation).

Physical Examination and Pathophysiology

In the absence of pericardial disease, diastolic pressure is determined by the cardiac chamber's compliance (or "stretchability"). Thus, the thick-walled left ventricle has a higher diastolic pressure than the thin-walled, more compliant right ventricle. With pericardial tamponade, pressure in the pericardial space, normally near zero, increases and exceeds diastolic pressure in the cardiac chambers. Diastolic pressure in the heart is then governed by pressure outside the heart, and for this reason the LV and right ventricular (RV) diastolic pressures become identical. Essentially the same thing happens with constriction; as the heart fills during diastole, the chambers "hit the wall" of scarred pericardium, and this determines diastolic pressure.

In both cases, hemodynamics makes the diagnosis: Simultaneous LV and RV diastolic pressures are identical (Fig. 7.3). With constriction, the sudden limitation of early diastolic filling ("hitting the wall") also produces a dip-and-plateau or "square root" pattern.

Pulsus Paradoxus This physical finding is more prominent with tamponade than constriction. In truth, there is nothing paradoxical about it. Normally the systolic blood pressure falls less than 10 mm Hg during inspiration, and with pulsus paradoxus it falls more. In extreme cases it falls enough that there is a perceptible reduction in pulse volume with inspiration.

The physiology of "pulsus" is complex. Intrathoracic pressure becomes negative during inspiration, sucking blood (as well as air) into the chest and increasing venous return to the right heart. RV volume increases, and the expanded right ventricle pushes the interventricular septum toward the left ventricle, reducing LV volume. In addition, pulmonary venous return to the left atrium is decreased during inspiration. Physiologists describe this as "respiratory preload variation" (RV preload rises and LV preload falls). The net effect is a reduction in LV stroke volume and of systolic blood pressure.

Tamponade and constriction cause an exaggeration of these changes. Both ventricles are smaller than usual because of elevated pericardial pressure. With inspiration there is still a drop in intrathoracic pressure and an increase in flow to the right ventricle. Bowing of the septum toward the left ventricle has an even greater effect because of reduced LV size. The reduction in LV stroke volume is accentuated, leading to an even greater drop in systolic blood pressure during inspiration.

Pulsus is measured with the patient breathing normally. The best method is to inflate the blood pressure cuff and then have it deflate very, very (very) slowly. You will initially hear the Korotkoff sounds during expiration but not during inspiration; record that blood pressure as the "expiratory pressure." As the cuff

FIGURE 7.3. Simultaneous left and right ventricular (LV and RV) pressures in a patient with constrictive pericarditis. Normally, the left ventricular pressure is much higher than right ventricular pressure during diastole, and identical pressure during diastole is a hallmark of both constriction and pericardial tamponade. In addition, this patient has the early diastolic pressure dip and then plateau that is typical of constriction (best seen in the first and last beats). (Reproduced by permission from Kern MJ. The cardiac catheterization handbook. St. Louis, MO: Mosby, 1999:203.)

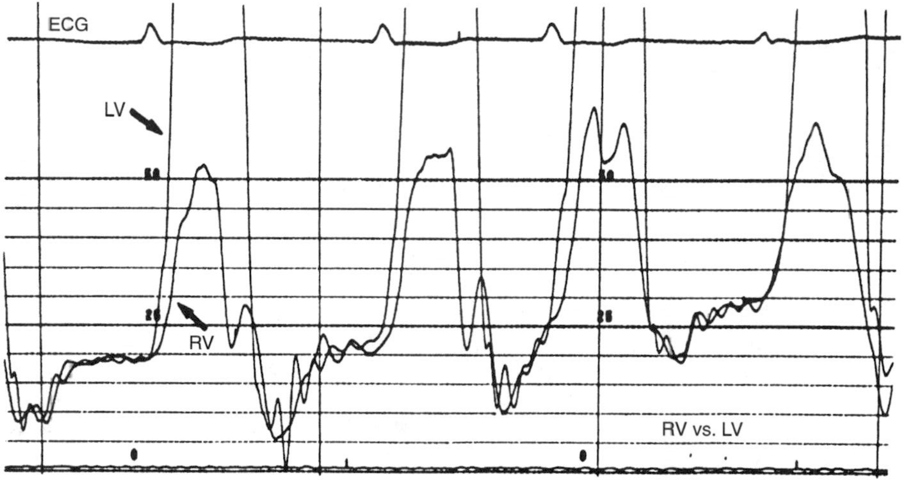

continues to deflate slowly, at some point you will begin to hear the sounds during inspiration and expiration (throughout the respiratory cycle); record that pressure measurement as the "inspiratory pressure." The difference between these first and second pressure measurements quantifies the pulsus paradoxus.

Other Physical Findings and Laboratory Examination The jugular venous pulse is elevated with both tamponade and constriction. With constriction there may also be an inspiratory increase rather than the normal fall in jugular venous pulse (Kussmaul's sign). A diastolic pericardial knock soon after S_2 may be audible with constriction (possibly the heart "hitting the wall").

The ECG may show diffuse ST elevation when there is acute pericarditis. Later, T waves may invert, but before they do the STs become isoelectric. This distinguishes the ST-T changes of pericarditis from those of myocardial infarction, where T waves invert while the ST segments are still elevated. In most cases of tamponade and constriction, ST elevation is not present. QRS voltage may be low when large effusion provides "insulation." There may be electrical alternans, a rise and fall in QRS voltage, as the heart swings in the enlarged pericardial space.

Pericardial calcification on chest x-ray supports a clinical diagnosis of constriction. Get an overpenetrated chest x-ray to look for it. Magnetic resonance imaging has been reported to show thickened pericardium, but I have never seen the test help make or exclude the diagnosis.

The echocardiogram detects even small effusions. With tamponade there may be apparent "collapse" of the atria. In some cases the pericardium appears thickened when there is constriction, but like magnetic resonance imaging, the echocardiogram cannot reliably make or exclude the diagnosis. When constriction is suspected, simultaneous measurement of RV and LV pressure in the catheterization laboratory is needed.

In addition to blood tests to diagnose conditions that may cause pericardial effusion (not reviewed here), diagnostic pericardiocentesis may help. Cytology is usually positive when the effusion is malignant (and the fluid is often bloody).

Cor Pulmonale

Lung disease can cause pulmonary hypertension, leading to right heart failure ("cor pulmonale"). The three mechanisms are hypoxic vasoconstriction (especially chronic bronchitis, cystic fibrosis, obesity hypoventilation, and other hypoventilation syndromes), obstruction of the pulmonary vascular bed (pulmonary embolism, primary pulmonary hypertension, sickle cell disease), and obliteration of lung parenchyma with loss of vascular surface area (emphysema, bronchiectasis, cystic fibrosis, interstitial lung disease).

Hypoxia is a potent pulmonary vasoconstrictor. When prolonged, there is an increase in the thickness of the walls of small pulmonary artery (PA) branches and, eventually, irreversible fibrosis. A patient with chronic obstructive pulmonary disease and hypoxia, the "blue bloater" with chronic bronchitis, is more prone to cor pulmonale than others with emphysema and equally severe airway obstruction but with normal arterial oxygen saturation (the "pink puffer"). One indication for home oxygen therapy is relief of pulmonary hypertension in those with hypoxemia and right heart failure.

Clinical Presentation

The clinical syndrome is right heart failure—lower extremity edema—in a patient with lung disease, no pulmonary congestion, and normal LV function. Dyspnea is usual but is caused by the lung disease. Palpitations and atrial arrhythmias are common, especially multifocal atrial tachycardia (Fig. 7.4).

The cardiac findings with RV failure are subtle. There may be an accentuated P_2, indicating pulmonary hypertension. You may hear a right-sided S_3 gallop (audible during inspiration). There may be an RV lift and jugular venous distention with a prominent A wave. If there is a large V wave, consider tricuspid regurgitation as a complication of pulmonary hypertension. With RV failure, there may be an inspiratory rise in jugular venous pressure (Kussmaul's sign).

Although the pulmonary examination is abnormal with chronic obstructive pulmonary disease, a normal examination does not exclude cor pulmonale. Other causes such as primary pulmonary hypertension, recurrent pulmonary embolus, or sleep apnea may not change the lung examination.

Laboratory Examination

The chest x-ray findings of pulmonary hypertension and cor pulmonale are enlargement of the right ventricle and the central

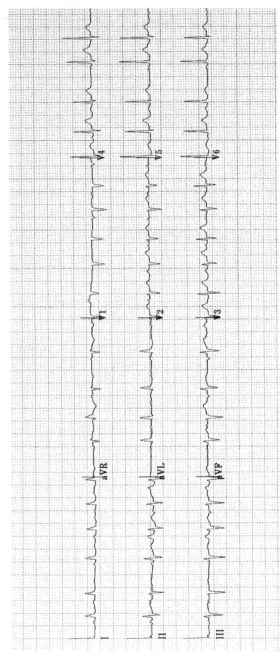

FIGURE 7.4. Multifocal atrial tachycardia. The rhythm is irregular, and there is variable P wave morphology. (Reproduced by permission from Taylor GJ. 150 Practice ECGs. Cambridge, MA: Blackwell Science, 1997.)

TABLE 7.3. Diagnosis of RV Hypertrophy

Criteria
R/S in $V_1 \geq 1$, *or*
R in $V_1 \geq 7$ mm, *or*
R in V_1 + S in V_5 or V_6 > 10.5 mm

Supportive findings
Right axis deviation > 110 degrees
Right atrial abnormality
ST depression + T wave inversion in V_1 or V_2 (RV strain)

pulmonary arteries. A lack of vessel markings at the periphery of the lung fields in contrast to the large central vessels produces a "pruned tree" appearance.

The ECG is a nonspecific test. There may be right ventricular hypertrophy or P pulmonale (Table 7.3 and Figure 7.5), but an absence of RV hypertrophy on the ECG does not exclude cor pulmonale. Low QRS voltage is common with emphysema, as is delay in R wave progression. Atrial arrhythmias, including atrial flutter, fibrillation, and multifocal atrial tachycardia, are common. Successful treatment of lung disease tends to improve arrhythmia control.

The echocardiogram is the key test, because it allows evaluation of RV and right atrial size (you will get a qualitative assessment, not a numerical size). Both are enlarged with cor pulmonale. RV wall thickness is difficult to measure, so the echo is not reliable for the diagnosis of RV hypertrophy. Mild tricuspid regurgitation is common when there is pulmonary hypertension. PA pressure can be estimated using Doppler techniques. The echocardiogram is also useful for excluding nonpulmonary causes of pulmonary hypertension, such as occult mitral stenosis. In many patients with advanced lung disease, especially emphysema, cardiac structures may be difficult to visualize. The transesophageal echo is an alternative but is slightly higher risk for patients with obstructive lung disease. The clinical diagnosis of cor pulmonale usually is sufficient, and transesophageal echo is unnecessary.

The central hemodynamic event in cor pulmonale is elevated PA pressure. The pulmonary wedge pressure is normal unless there is LV dysfunction. Normally, the PA diastolic pressure is equal to the pulmonary wedge pressure (during diastole the PA, left atrium, and LV are in open communication). With an increase in pulmonary vascular resistance (PVR), there is a

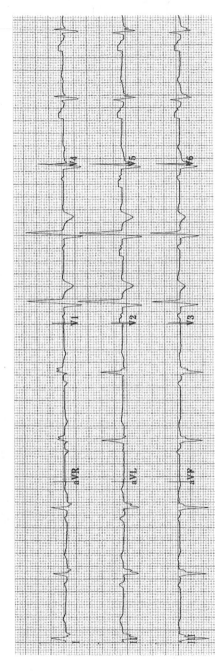

FIGURE 7.5. RV hypertrophy. There is a tall R wave in V₁, deep S wave in V₆, and ST-T wave changes in the right precordial leads (the RV strain pattern). Taller P waves in II, III, and aVF would indicate right atrial abnormality (see Table 7.3 and Practice ECG A3). (Reproduced by permission from Taylor GJ. 150 Practice ECGs. Cambridge, MA: Blackwell Science, 1997.)

gradient between PA diastolic and left atrial pressure (this is called the transpulmonary gradient). PVR is elevated with cor pulmonale. I have said that cor pulmonale is pulmonary hypertension in the face of normal LV diastolic pressures. It is possible to have cor pulmonale plus LV failure, as smokers often develop left heart disease. In such cases the pulmonary wedge pressure (left atrial pressure) is high, but the PA diastolic pressure is even higher. This transpulmonary gradient defines elevated PVR, the constant finding of cor pulmonale.

A variety of other tests may be needed to determine the etiology. When there is no apparent lung disease, recurrent pulmonary embolus may be confirmed with perfusion scanning or angiography. A sleep study may be needed to diagnose sleep apnea. Serologic testing for inflammatory lung disorders may be considered. Lung biopsy is occasionally needed to diagnose pulmonary fibrosis, connective tissue disease, or primary pulmonary hypertension. The history and physical examination help focus the workup.

Treatment

Improving oxygenation relieves pulmonary vasoconstriction, and cor pulmonale is an indication for home oxygen therapy. The goal is to keep the PaO_2 above 60 mm Hg. Supplemental oxygen must be used cautiously when there is chronic hypercarbia and respiratory acidosis. Vigorous treatment of the lung disease is critical.

Specific treatment of the heart failure is of limited benefit. Severe edema requires diuretic therapy. When there is splanchnic congestion, consider using the loop diuretics that are best absorbed (torsemide and bumetanide rather than furosemide; see Chapter 1). Vasodilator therapy has little effect on PVR when there is parenchymal lung disease, and "afterload reduction therapy" is not indicated. Primary pulmonary hypertension may respond to intravenous prostacyclin.

Digoxin is not helpful for the treatment of right heart failure and is of limited benefit in controlling ventricular rate when there are atrial tachyarrhythmias. Multifocal atrial tachycardia tends not to respond, and those with cor pulmonale are more susceptible to digitalis toxicity. For these reasons, verapamil is a better choice for rate control.

Successful treatment of atrial tachyarrhythmias, like heart failure, usually requires control of the lung disease. Membrane active antiarrhythmic agents are generally ineffective, and rate control is difficult. Cardioversion may be considered, but maintaining sinus rhythm is unlikely unless pulmonary function is improved.

Eisenmenger's Syndrome

Adults who are cyanotic and have a history of congenital heart disease often have Eisenmenger's syndrome, with pulmonary hypertension and possibly right heart failure. The most common causes are ventricular septal defect (VSD), patent ductus arteriosus (PDA), and transposition of the great vessels. The size of the shunt is the key factor in developing pulmonary hypertension. About half of those with large VSD or PDA develop Eisenmenger's syndrome.

Lesions that transmit both high volume and pressure to the PA more commonly provoke pulmonary hypertension, explaining why VSD and PDA are common causes. With these high-pressure lesions, pulmonary hypertension becomes fixed in infancy. Atrial septal defect (ASD), which delivers high volume but not pressure to the PA, may rarely cause Eisenmenger's syndrome. In such cases, it develops later in life.

High pulmonary blood flow and pressure lead to irreversible microvascular changes. Why some patients have vascular injury while others do not is uncertain. Endothelial dysfunction, growth factors, and platelet aggregation contribute to intimal proliferation and progressive occlusion of small arterioles. With these anatomic changes, high PVR is irreversible.

Eventually, pulmonary resistance exceeds systemic resistance. The direction of shunting reverses, becoming right to left. Desaturated blood reaches the left heart, and the resulting arterial hypoxemia stimulates erythrocytosis.

Clinical Presentation and Management

Most patients have symptoms of low cardiac output, including fatigue and poor exercise tolerance. Right heart failure is common, and there may be an element of left heart congestion as well. The patient's appearance is striking, with central cyanosis and clubbed fingers. The cardiac examination reflects the underlying condition.

Erythrocytosis causing hyperviscosity is the major day-to-day management issue. Formerly we used frequent phlebotomy to keep the hematocrit under 65%. Targeting the hematocrit is not the current practice. Rather, the indication for phlebotomy is symptoms of hyperviscosity, including headache, irritability, lethargy, fatigue, dizziness, and visual disturbances. Most develop symptoms when the hematocrit approaches 70%, and the goal of phlebotomy is to reduce it below 65%. Simultaneous volume replacement with saline is needed.

Iron deficiency and microcytosis are common, especially with recurrent phlebotomy. The small red blood cells are rigid, do not deform normally, do not pass through capillaries as easily and aggravate sludging. When red cell indices indicate microcytosis or there is low serum iron, iron therapy is needed (an apparent paradox in a patient with an elevated hematocrit).

There are a number of other complications of Eisenmenger's syndrome. With right-left shunting, paradoxical embolus is a possible cause of stroke. For the same reason, brain abscess may be a consequence of transient bacteremia. Stress is poorly tolerated. With pregnancy, maternal mortality is about 45%, and pregnancy is inadvisable. The perioperative mortality is high with noncardiac surgery. High altitude travel should be avoided, and commercial air transportation is best tolerated with the patient on supplemental oxygen.

Clinical Course

The prognosis with Eisenmenger's syndrome is better than it is with other causes of pulmonary hypertension. Survival is 80% at 10 years, 77% at 15 years, and 42% at 25 years. Predictors of early mortality include syncope, elevated RV filling pressure and right heart failure, and more severe hypoxemia (oxygen saturation less than 85% at rest). The location of the right-to-left shunt does not affect prognosis. The causes of death include ventricular fibrillation, heart failure, hemoptysis, stroke, brain abscess, thromboembolism, and complications of surgery or pregnancy.

ATRIAL SEPTAL DEFECT

There are three possible sites of communication between the right and left atria. The most common defect (more than 80% of cases) is the ostium secundum ASD, located in the mid-septum, well above the atrioventricular valves.

The ostium primum defect (15% of cases) originates in the endocardial cushion, a structure in the center of the fetal heart that also contributes to the formation of the mitral and tricuspid valves and the upper part of the interventricular septum. The most extreme form of endocardial cushion defect is the absence of these structures, resulting in a single-chambered heart. With primum ASD, there may be cleft mitral or tricuspid leaflets and regurgitation. The interventricular conduction system also is affected, and left axis deviation (usually left anterior fascicular block) is a marker of primum ASD. The sinus venosus defect is the least common ASD, occurring at the entrance of either the superior or the inferior vena cava.

The usual ASD is large, often 2 cm in diameter. Because of its size, there is no jet effect and little turbulence. Thus, the ASD itself does not generate a murmur. The large defect also means that pressures in the two atria are equal. Blood flows toward the right atrium because the right ventricle is more compliant than the left ventricle during diastole.

The major hemodynamic effects are RA, RV, and PA volume overload. When the catheterization report indicates a 2:1 shunt, it means that the pulmonary blood flow is twice the systemic blood flow and that the right ventricle is handling twice as much volume as the left ventricle. Increased pulmonary blood flow may provoke a rise in PA pressure, and a form of Eisenmenger's syndrome occurs in about 10% of patients, usually in adolescence. The incidence of Eisenmenger's reaction with VSD or PDA is higher and the onset is younger. These conditions increase flow to the PA, but they also transmit systemic pressure (either LV or aortic systolic pressure) to the PA. The combination of high pressure and high flow is a stronger stimulus of pulmonary vascular reactivity.

Clinical Presentation, Laboratory Evaluation, and Treatment

ASD is often diagnosed late in life. Children and young adults are asymptomatic, and the diagnosis is made with routine physical examination or chest x-ray. Middle-aged patients usually present with atrial arrhythmias. Heart failure may develop as the initial symptom in older people. It would seem that the left ventricle would be protected, but a common pattern is biventricular failure and not isolated RV failure.

This probably has to do with how the interventricular septum works. It has to "choose sides," to work as a part of either the left or right ventricle. It chooses the side with the greater workload, normally the left ventricle. With chronic RV overload, it works instead with the right ventricle, moving away from the lateral wall of the left ventricle rather than toward it during systole. This is the so-called paradoxical septal motion described by the echocardiogram when there is RV overload. Loss of septal function may contribute to the eventual failure of the left ventricle when there is chronic RV overload. In this case, "chronic" may mean five to six decades of abnormal cardiac loading before symptoms develop.

The physical findings of ASD are obvious. S_2 is widely split, with no respiratory variation. Because of volume overload, emptying of the right ventricle is delayed, and P_2 is late. The large ASD distributes the increased venous return to the heart during inspiration equally to both atria. Fixed splitting of S_2 is a reliable finding, and its absence excludes ASD.

There is usually a systolic murmur at the left base. This is not caused by flow across the ASD but rather by high flow across the normal pulmonic valve (with a 2:1 shunt, the pulmonic valve has twice the normal flow). With a primum defect, a cleft mitral or tricuspid leaflet causes the typical regurgitant murmur.

The typical pattern of RV volume overload on the ECG is incomplete right bundle branch block, a usual finding with ASD. The primum defect usually causes left anterior fascicular block, and checking the axis in a patient with ASD is a mark of clinical sophistication. Pulmonary plethora on the chest x-ray is always present, and experienced radiologists claim that it is not subtle (though I have a hard time seeing it). *A normal chest x-ray and ECG exclude significant right-left shunting and ASD.* The echocardiogram is not needed to exclude ASD.

When ASD is present the echocardiogram confirms RV enlargement and paradoxical septal motion. The ASD is easily visualized, and flow across the defect is documented with echocardiographic contrast agents and Doppler. In addition, the echo-Doppler study allows estimation of PA pressure.

Surgical repair of ASD is recommended when the pulmonary to systemic blood flow is above 1.5:1, especially when the RV size is increased. Surgery is not done to prevent pulmonary hypertension, a rare complication that develops before age 30 when it does occur. In middle age, repair is done to prevent atrial arrhythmias and eventual heart failure. There is a survival benefit with surgery even for patients older than 50 years, most of whom are symptomatic.

Because there is no jet effect, endocarditis prophylaxis is not indicated for ASD.

END-OF-LIFE DECISIONS AND PALLIATIVE CARE FOR PATIENTS WITH HEART DISEASE

You will observe a general reluctance to "give up" on the patient with heart disease. It is not quite like cancer, and there is always the possibility of one more interventional procedure. Scientific medicine's central ethic is prolongation of life, and aggressive therapy often is life saving. But there is a dilemma when life-prolonging surgery seems too aggressive for an elderly or severely disabled person. This is especially true for the patient who has had multiple cardiac procedures in the past.

A first step in resolving the dilemma is considering the patient's wishes. The "new medical ethics" that has evolved in recent decades is based on patient autonomy. As doctors we do not have unquestioned control over what happens to patients. Instead, our responsibility is to inform, recommend alternatives, and then to respect and support the patient's decision. This means that when we are old and sick no one can make us do something we do not want. It is what we want for ourselves, and it should be what we want for our patients.

Even so, surveys of elderly patients and their families document concern about inappropriate and aggressive care at the end of life. Old people often believe that they are convinced to have procedures they do not want.

Peaceful Death, Another Goal of Medicine

In addition to prolonging life and relieving suffering, at some stage of our lives another goal of medical care is a peaceful death. We wince at the spectacle of the hopelessly ill old person subjected to the savagery of a prolonged intensive care unit death.

The trend in scientific medicine has been the elimination of illnesses that are rapidly fatal. What remain are conditions like dementia, stroke, and heart failure. I am now encountering chronically ill elderly people who have decided to reclaim the traditional "old man's friends" by declining curative treatment for acute illnesses such as pneumonia, heart attack, or urosepsis. They usually meet resistance from their doctors. However, an autonomous person has the right to refuse any treatment, whether it is chemotherapy for advanced cancer, antibiotics for pneumonia, or surgery for aortic stenosis.

This is not an argument against life-prolonging therapy for old people. Indeed, treatment shown to prolong life by clinical trials should be applied irrespective of age, *if that is what the patient wants*. Instead, you should support your patient who has decided to avoid possibly life-prolonging but *unwanted* therapy.

If you do, are you are in some way responsible for your patient's death? If you believe that, you have fallen prey to the doctor's delusion of control over life and death. In matter of fact, a terminally ill patient dies of a disease. Our intervention affects only the timing and the amount of suffering. By avoiding life-prolonging therapy at the patient's direction, the doctor is not responsible for death nor is the patient. (Daniel Callahan develops this line of reasoning in *The Troubled Dream of Life*, and I recommend it to you and your patients.)

Palliative Care

Even those with terminal heart failure and CAD should have aggressive medical therapy, because it controls symptoms. When usual drug therapies become ineffective, it is time add hospice care.

Current federal regulations provide for hospice care if survival is estimated to be less than 6 months, and patients with advanced heart disease meet this criterion. Hospice nurses are good at regulating heart failure therapy, including the use of intravenous diuretics and even dobutamine. Such measures may enable the patient to remain at home, out of the hospital.

Morphine

Morphine is the key addition to end-stage care when standard therapy no longer controls symptoms. As a venodilator, it reduces blood return to the heart and relieves pulmonary congestion. In addition, it blunts the anxiety that comes with severe dyspnea.

There is concern that morphine may depress respiration. In practice, with all but extreme doses, this is rare for patients with pulmonary edema (or with severe dyspnea in advanced lung disease).

Oral morphine (Roxanol) may control symptoms, and it can be supplemented with a nebulized preparation. Parenteral morphine is more difficult to administer in the outpatient setting. Hospice nurses have experience with the drug—more than most physicians—and can competently regulate even parenteral use for patients with heart failure or intractable angina. A brief inpatient stay may help with determining the effective dose.

Rest Therapy

Another option for those with uncontrolled angina is reduced activity, a "bed-to-chair" lifestyle. This was a common approach before the 1960s, and at times it is still appropriate. I am a strong believer in the value of exercise therapy for CAD, but there comes a time when it does not work, and reduced activity offers palliation. Some elderly patients prefer this alternative to open heart surgery.

Extreme Symptoms in the Terminal Patient

What do we do for a patient with end-stage disease who comes to the emergency room with extreme symptoms? A common issue is pulmonary edema unresponsive to intravenous diuretics. It is unfortunate when the doctor offers intubation and ventilation as the only hope for relieving symptoms. Despite a previous decision to avoid ventilator therapy, a desperate patient and family may have a change of mind when this seems the only chance for relief.

An effective alternative is higher dose morphine, titrated to relieve dyspnea. There may be depression of respiration with a dose sufficient to relieve symptoms. In this case the moral imperative is to provide relief of suffering for the dying patient, even if high-dose opiates contribute to more rapid death. There is no culpability. This is not assisted suicide or euthanasia but rather necessary therapy for extreme symptoms.

SUGGESTED READINGS
Preoperative Evaluation

American College of Physicians. Guidelines for assessing and managing the perioperative risk from coronary artery disease associated with major non cardiac surgery. Ann Intern Med 1997;127: 309–313.

Eagle KA, Brundage, BH, Chaitman BR, et al. Guidelines for perioperative cardiovascular evaluation for non cardiac surgery: report of the American College of Cardiology. American Heart Association Task Force. J Am Coll Cardiol 1996;27:910–926.

Eagle KA, Coley CM, Newell JB, et al. Combining clinical and thallium data optimizes preoperative assessment of cardiac risk before major vascular surgery. Ann Intern Med 1989;110:859–866.

Mangano DT, Layug EL, Wallace A, Tareo I. Effects of atenolol on mortality and cardiovascular morbidity after non-cardiac surgery. The Multicenter Study of Perioperative Ischemia Research Group. N Engl J Med 1996;335:1713–1719.

Palda VA, Detsky AS. Perioperative assessment and management of risk from coronary artery disease. Ann Intern Med 1997;127:313–318.

Smetana GW. Preoperative pulmonary evaluation. N Engl J Med 1999;340:937–944. (Not the subject of this chapter, but it rounds out the preoperative evaluation. History and physical examination are as important as spirometry in predicting respiratory failure and ventilator dependence.)

Vanzetto G, Machecourt J, Blendea D, et al. Additive value of thallium myocardial imaging for prediction of perioperative events in clinically selected high cardiac risk patient having abdominal aortic surgery. Am J Cardiol 1996;77:143–150.

Systemic Congestion and Isolated Right Heart Failure

Ammash N, Warnes CA. Cerebrovascular events in adult patients with cyanotic congenital heart disease. J Am Coll Cardiol 1996;28:768–775.

Brickner ME, Hillis LD, Lange RA. Congenital heart disease in adults. N Engl J Med 2000;342(Pt 1):256–263, 342(pt 2): 334–342.

Fishman AP. Pulmonary hypertension: beyond vasodilator therapy. N Engl J Med 1998;338:321–324.

Fishman AP, Palevsky HI. Pulmonary hypertension and chronic cor pulmonale. Heart Dis Stroke 1993;2:335–341.

Mehta A, Mehta M, Jain AC. Constrictive pericarditis. Clin Cardiol 1999;22:334–344.

Myers RB, Spodick DH. Constrictive pericarditis: clinical and pathophysiologic characteristics. Am Heart J 1999;138:219–232.

Tsang TS, Oh JK, Seward JB. Diagnosis and management of cardiac tamponade in the era of echocardiography. Clin Cardiol 1999;22:446–452.

VongpatanasinW, Brickner ME, Hillis LD, Lang RA. The Eisenmenger syndrome in adults. Ann Intern Med 1998;128: 745–751.

White J, Bullock RE, Hudgson P, Gibson FJ. Neuromuscular disease, respiratory failure and cor pulmonale. Postgrad Med J 1992;68:820–826.

Wiedemann HP, Matthay RA. Cor pulmonale in chronic obstructive pulmonary disease: circulatory pathophysiology and management. Clin Chest Med 1990;11:523–531.

End-of-Life Decisions and Palliative Care

Callahan D. The troubled dream of life. New York, Simon and Schuster, 1993.

Johnson-Neely K, Crammer LM. End-of-life care: palliative strategies for vomiting and dyspnea. Fam Pract Recert 1998; 20:13–22. (Addresses the goal of therapy for the patient with extreme symptoms, and the risk of respiratory depression.)

King SB III, Ullyot DJ, Basta L, et al. Application of medical and surgical interventions near the end of life. J Am Coll Cardiol 1998;31:933–939.

Lentzner H, Pamuk E, Rhodenhiser E, et al. The quality of life in the year before death. Am J Public Health 1992;82:1093–1099.

Lynn J, Teno J, Phillips R, et al. Perceptions by family members of the dying experience of older and seriously ill patients. Ann Intern Med 1997;126:97–103.

Sachs GA, Ahronheim J, Rhymes J, et al. Good care of dying patients: the alternative to physician-assisted suicide and euthanasia. J Am Geriatr Soc 1995;43:553–560.

Practice Electrocardiograms

Note: read these as unknowns. The clinical issues have been covered in the text, and this ECG reading exercise is another self-test.

Abbreviations you will encounter in the ECG reading station:

AF	atrial fibrillation
AV & AVB	atrio-ventricular, AV block
BBB	bundle branch block
LAA, LAE	left atrial abnormality (enlargement)
LAD	left axis deviation
LAFB	left anterior fascicular block
LBBB	left bundle branch block
LPFB	left posterior fascicular block
LV & LVH	left ventricle (ventricular), LV hypertrophy
MI	myocardial infarction
NSR	normal sinus rhythm
NSSTTWC	nonspecific ST-T wave changes
NSSTC	nonspecific ST segment changes
PAC	premature atrial contraction
PRWP	poor R wave progresssion
PSVT	paroxysmal supraventricular tachycardia
PVC, PVB	premature ventricular contraction (beat)
RAA, RAE	right atrial abnormality (enlargement)
RAD	right axis deviation
RBBB	right bundle branch block
RV, RVH	right ventricule (ventricular), RV hypertrophy
SEMI	subendocardial MI (a.k.a. non-Q wave MI)
ST	sinus tachycardia
VPB	ventricular premature beat (a.k.a. PVC)
VT, VF	ventricular tachycardia (fibrillation)
WPW	Wolff-Parkinson-White syndrome

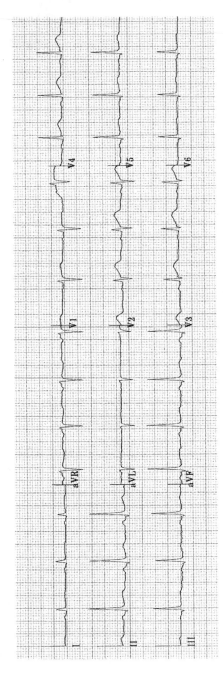

FIGURE A.1. 36-year-old man; life insurance examination, no history of heart disease.

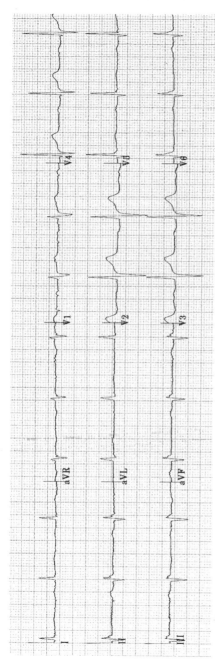

FIGURE A.2. 76-year-old man with history of MI and mild heart failure. Does this ECG tell you anything about the patient's coronary anatomy?

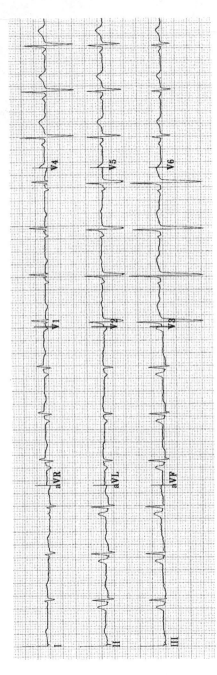

FIGURE A.3. 59-year-old woman with peripheral edema, jugular venous distension, and a loud systolic murmur that intensifies with inspiration.

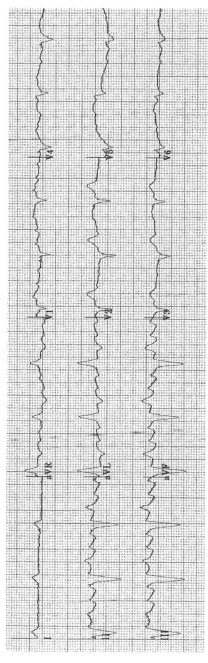

FIGURE A.4. 70-year-old man with a remote history of fainting spells. Now in the emergency room with dyspnea and fever.

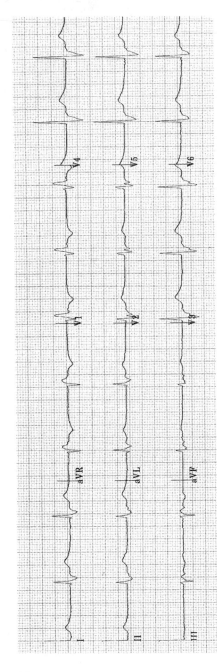

FIGURE A.5. 80-year-old man treated with diuretics and digoxin. What lab work is needed?

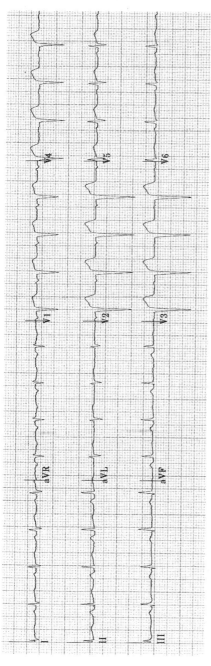

FIGURE A.6. 52-year-old man who had a 20-hour siege of indigestion a month earlier. He has severe fatigue. The cardiologist has ordered an echocardiogram. Why?

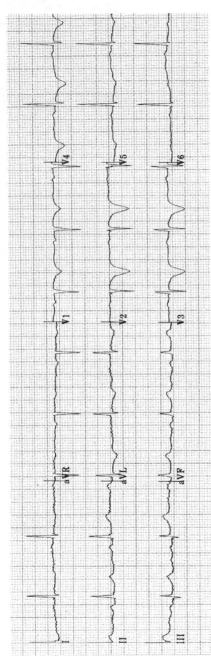

FIGURE A.7. 71-year-old woman in the emergency room. A long episode of chest pain was relieved before her arrival by nitroglycerin. Is angiography indicated? What would it show?

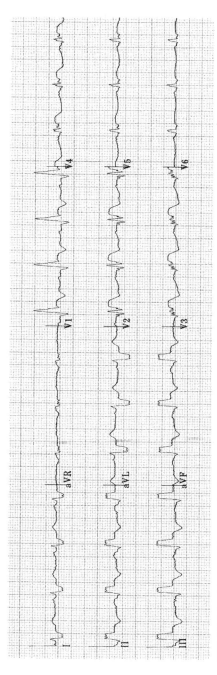

FIGURE A.8. 85-year-old man with chest pain. There is a history of prior MI. What is his prognosis?

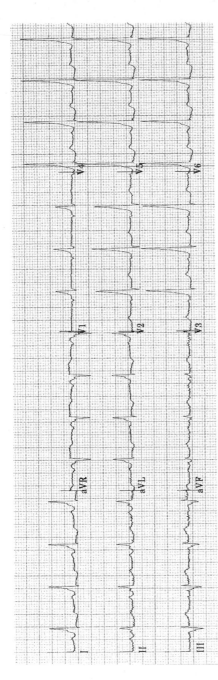

FIGURE A.9. 42-year-old man with intermittent palpitations since childhood. His doctor is concerned about his conduction abnormality and a silent heart attack.

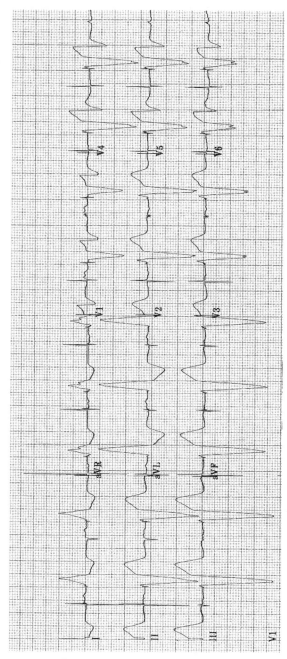

FIGURE A.10. 73-year-old man; no history provided.

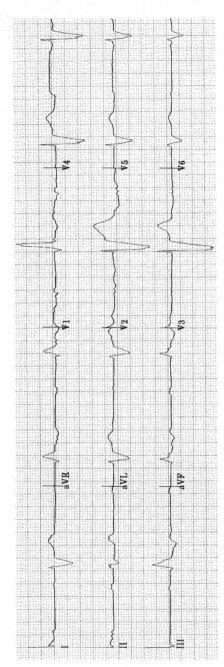

FIGURE A.11. 82-year-old man with fatigue and ankle edema for 2 weeks.

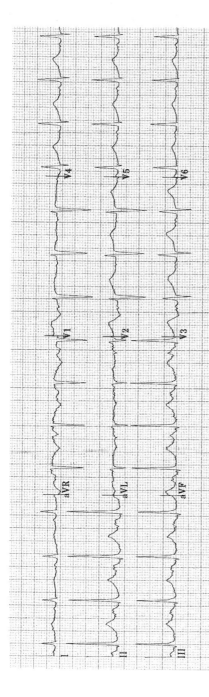

FIGURE A.12. 40-year-old man in the emergency room following an episode of syncope. He has been treated with erythromycin and antihistamines for a respiratory illness.

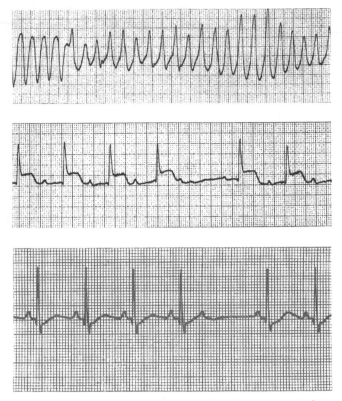

FIGURE A.13. Top: Telemetry recording from the same patient (no. 12) 4 hours later. During the arrhythmia, he lost consciousness. Middle: 68-year-old woman with acute inferior MI. Does she need a temporary pacemaker? Bottom: A patient with an irregular pulse.

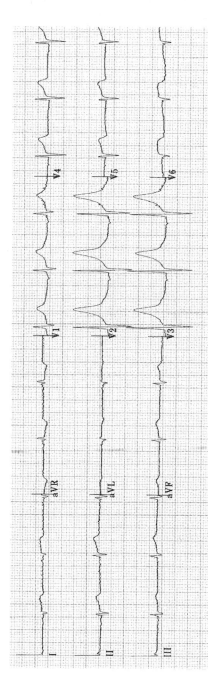

FIGURE A.14. 46-year-old man with 3 hours of chest pain. What is the treatment?

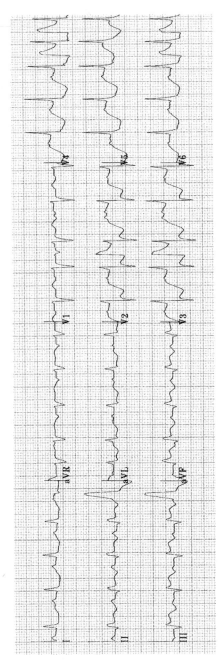

FIGURE A.15. 74-year-old man in the emergency room with chest pain that began 30 minutes ago. Is this angina or MI? Is the ischemia anterior or inferior?

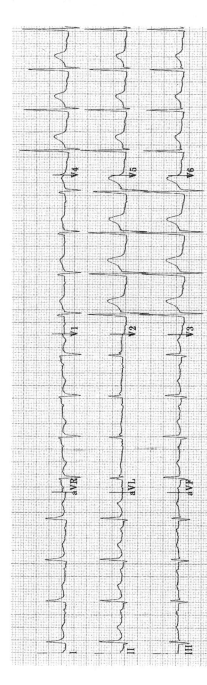

FIGURE A.16. 54-year-old man with no history of heart disease. He weighs 275 pounds.

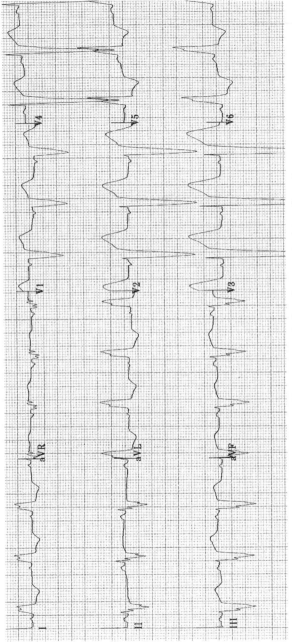

FIGURE A.17. 67-year-old woman with a history of hypertension. Is there hypertensive heart disease?

A.1. *I: NSR 80 beats/min. PR 0.12, QRS 0.09, QT normal. Axis 80°. Probably normal ECG with small inferior Q's noted and diffuse J-point elevation (consider early repolarization).*

C: For a Q wave to be significant, it should be a box deep and a box wide. These inferior Q waves do not make it; I mention them to make it clear they were not overlooked.

The *J point* is the junction between the QRS and the ST segment. In this case, it is above the baseline in V_2 through V_6, and minimally so in inferior and lateral leads. The ST segments are elevated but maintain normal shape with upward concavity. This ST elevation is worth mention, but it should be interpreted in clinical context. For a patient in the emergency room with chest pain, it could indicate pericarditis (it involves multiple vascular distributions, and normal upward concavity is maintained); you could not be sure from this tracing. Because you know that this is an insurance examination and he is young, early repolarization is a safe guess (and it is identified as a guess on the report).

A.2. *I: NSR 70 beats/min. PR 0.24, QRS 0.09, QT normal. Axis –30°. Abnormal due to 1° AVB, LAD, and inferolateral MI of uncertain age.*

C: When compared with the previous case, this patient's Q waves are deeper and wider and are found in all three of the inferior leads. The diagnosis of inferior MI is certain. There are also deep Q waves in V_5 and V_6, lateral leads. Perhaps he has had two MIs with occlusion of the artery to the inferior wall, then occlusion of another vessel to the lateral wall. But this is unlikely. Instead, the coronary artery supplying this patient's inferior wall probably was large, wrapping around the heart and supplying a part of the lateral wall as well. The resulting infarct was large enough to leave him with heart failure. Inferior MI is usually smaller and less consequential than anterior infarction; this case may be an exception.

A.3. *I: NSR 80 beats/min. PR 0.13, QRS 0.09, QT normal. Axis 100°. Abnormal due to biatrial abnormality, PRWP, and right ventricular hypertrophy.*

C: RAA is obvious (tall P waves in inferior leads); LAA is arguable, as there is no positive deflection before the negative deflection in V_1. RVH—tall R in V_1, deep S in V_6, T inversion in V_1 (the strain pattern), RAD, RAA. Based on physical findings and the ECG, the patient probably has tricuspid regurgitation.

A.4. *I: Atrial flutter and a ventricular pacemaker at 70 beats/min.*

C: The sawtooth flutter waves are apparent in the inferior leads. Look at the QRS complexes in I and II; there is a small pacing spike at the beginning of each. The pacer must be located in the right ventricle, as there is a LBBB pattern. The QRS morphology of the paced beat is not usually mentioned in the formal interpretation.

A demand ventricular pacemaker is commonly set to pace at about 70 beats/min. It is designated a VVI pacemaker: ventricular sensing, ventricular pacing, and programmed to be inhibited from pacing if it senses a native QRS.

A.5. *I: Nodal rhythm, 58 beats/min. QRS 0.13, QT long for the rate. Axis about 10°. Abnormal due to a long QTc, rhythm, and RBBB.*

C: Retrograde P waves are seen at the beginning of the T wave in multiple leads. The QT seems quite long in V_4 and V_5, and the calculated QTc is 0.55 sec. Thiazide diuretics may depress potassium and/or magnesium levels, causing prolongation of the QT interval. It is important to diagnose and correct these electrolyte disturbances, as they may lead to ventricular arrhythmias and sudden death. Check a digoxin level as well, as the nodal rhythm may be evidence of digitalis toxicity.

A.6. *I: ST 108/min. PR 0.16, QRS 0.08, QT normal. Axis 70°. Abnormal due to ST, anterior MI of uncertain age with persistent ST elevation.*

C: Axis—close to isoelectric, though slightly negative, in aVL. He probably had the MI a month earlier and misinterpreted his symptoms. Resting tachycardia a month after anterior infarction is a worrisome finding, suggesting LV dysfunction. That is reason enough for an echocardiogram. In addition, persistent ST elevation in infarct zone leads may indicate an LV aneurysm. This unfortunate fellow should have had reperfusion therapy at the time of his acute MI.

A.7. *I: NSR 60 beats/min. PR 0.18, QRS 0.08, QT normal. Axis 45°. Abnormal due to deep T inversion in anterior leads consistent with ischemia or non-Q MI.*

C: She should be hospitalized and treated with aspirin, heparin, and antianginal drugs. Cardiac enzymes probably will be elevated, which would make the diagnosis of infarction rather than unstable angina. Angiography is indicated and probably would show a tight and ragged-appearing lesion in the anterior descending coronary artery, possibly with thrombus. Although this infarction is a small one, with only minimal injury to the anterior wall, she is at risk for occlusion and transmural MI.

A.8. *I: NSR 80 beats/min. PR 0.18, QRS 0.16, QT normal. Axis 100°. Abnormal due to RBBB, RAD, and possibly acute anterior and inferior MI.*

C: This is an unusual ECG because there is ST elevation in both inferior and anterior leads. Recall that it is uncommon for acute ischemia to occur simultaneously in two different vascular distributions. Why would two different arteries occlude at the same time? Global ST elevation instead suggests a global etiology such as pericarditis. But this looks more like ischemia to me, because the ST waves are upwardly convex, and because there is T inversion at the same time there is ST elevation. The T waves can invert with pericarditis, but the ST segments usually return to baseline before they do.

Here is more history that explains coincidental MIs. His right coronary artery occluded and he had inferior MI 2 years earlier, but the infarct was incomplete. He had collateral flow from the anterior descending artery to the distal right coronary artery. Although there was injury to the inferior wall, some muscle was saved by the collateral vessels. Now he has occluded the anterior descending artery, losing flow to the anterior wall plus the flow through the collaterals to his inferior wall. He is thus losing two vascular distributions with a single coronary occlusion. The prognosis is terrible.

This is an example of our ability to diagnose MI when there is RBBB.

A.9. *I: NSR 90 beats/min. PR 0.11, QRS 0.13, QT normal. Axis 15°. Abnormal due to preexcitation (WPW).*

C: The PR is borderline short (depends on the lead). There is a delta wave (lead I or the V leads). Compare this tracing with those demonstrating bundle branch block. With WPW, the *initial* portion of the QRS is slurred. With BBB, the *terminal* part of the QRS is slurred. This makes sense when you think of the pathophysiology of the two conditions. A blocked bundle branch causes a portion of the heart to be depolarized late, affecting the end of the QRS. There is a tall R wave in V_1 (consistent with posterior MI), and there are possible Q waves in inferior leads. Delta waves may appear as pseudo-Q waves.

A.10. *I: AV sequential pacemaker with 100% capture, 60 beats/min.*

C: There are pacing spikes before each P wave and QRS. The QRS has an LBBB pattern indicating a right ventricular location on the pacing electrode. This dual-chamber pacemaker, with leads in the right atrium and right ventricle, is called a DDD pacemaker: it has dual-chamber sensing, dual-chamber pacing, and dual sensing modes (pacing that can be either inhibited or triggered by preceding beats).

A.11. *I: Complete heart block, 36 beats/min. QRS 0.18, QT normal. Axis 130°. Abnormal due to the complete heart block and a ventricular escape rhythm.*

C: At first glance, I called this 2:1 AV block. With the Marquette equipment, the lead changes are instantaneous, and the top line of recording can be read as a continuous rhythm strip. Notice that the P waves that appear to be conducted (every other P wave) are followed by progressively longer PR intervals. The second-to-last beat has such a long PR that it is hard to believe the P is conducted. and the last beat has a short PR. Despite this variability of the PR, the ventricular rate is constant. The ventricular rate is not a multiple of the atrial rate; but it is close and for this reason has the appearance of 2:1 block. This is an example of AV dissociation and complete heart block.

The ventricular escape rhythm has a rate of 36 beats/min. This relatively rapid rhythm accounts for the absence of syncope. Why not diagnose RBBB + LPFB? The ventricular beats have that morphology, but they originate from the ventricle. The term *bundle branch block* indicates that the beat originates from above the bundle branch.

A.12. *I: NSR 90 beats/min. PR 0.18, QRS 0.09, QT is long for the rate with QTc 0.54. Axis 70°. Abnormal due to long QT and LAA*

C: There is notching of the P in lead II. The dominant finding is the long QT. Phenothiazine derivatives, including antihistamines, may lengthen the QT interval. When some antihistamines are combined with erythromycin, the QT interval prolongation may be aggravated; this combination may precipitate ventricular arrhythmias. The history of syncope and this ECG are indications for monitoring in the telemetry unit.

A.13 (top). *I: Polymorphic ventricular tachycardia, torsade de pointes.*
    C: Torsade de pointes is a form of VT that tends to occur with *conditions that prolong the QT interval.* Treatment of the arrhythmia includes measures that shorten the QT: magnesium infusion, increasing the heart rate with temporary pacing, or even isoproterenol infusion.

A.13 (middle). *I: The rhythm strip shows AV nodal Wenckebach (Mobitz I second-degree block).*
    C: There is progressive lengthening of the PR before the blocked beat, and the PR that follows the dropped beat is shorter.

A.13 (bottom). *I: Blocked PAC.*
    C: Look carefully at the T wave that precedes the pause. It is different from the other T waves, and the distortion is the ectopic P wave. Blocked PACs are commonly responsible for pauses and are diagnosed when distortion of the preceding T wave is recognized.

A.14. *I: NSR 65 beats/min. PR 0.12, QRS 0.08, QT long for the rate with QTc 0.56. Axis indeterminant. Abnormal due to posterolateral MI with acute lateral ischemia.*
    C: The QRS is isoelectric in multiple limb leads; if anything, the QRS vector is pointed back toward lead aVR. The tall R in V_1 is considered the equivalent of a posterior wall Q wave (perhaps you would see a Q with a V lead on the patient's back). Posterior or posterolateral MI may be caused by occlusion of the circumflex artery. There appears to be active ischemia, with persistent ST elevation and chest pain. An additional finding is tall peaked T waves in V_2 and V_3; these may be the hyperacute T waves of acute ischemia.
    The presence of Q waves does not mean that the MI is complete; continued pain and ST elevation just 3 hours from the onset of symptoms are indications for angioplasty or thrombolytic therapy.

A.15. *I: ST 120 beats/min. PR 0.18, QRS 0.10, QT long for the rate (QTc 0.50). Axis 30°. Abnormal due to acute inferior MI with reciprocal ST depression in anterolateral leads.*
    C: The ST elevation in the inferior leads is less prominent than the ST depression in anterolateral leads. Nevertheless, ST elevation defines the location of the MI. This patient had occlusion of a large right coronary artery, and the other vessels were normal. The presence of reciprocal ST depression identifies an inferior infarction as a large one. ST elevation and pain indicate transmural ischemia and infarction in progress, usually with (total) occlusion of the coronary artery.

A.16. *I: NSR 90 beats/min. PR 0.16, QRS 0.09, QT normal. Axis 30°. Borderline ECG due to possible inferior MI of uncertain age. Early repolarization noted.*

C: The Q waves are borderline. Early repolarization is not considered an abnormality. It is a common finding in thin young athletes (which this man is not). Roughly 10% to 15% of MIs are clinically silent. This patient needs further evaluation.

A.17. *I: NSR 80 beats/min. PR 0.14, QRS 0.14, QT long for the rate (QTc 0.50). Axis –60°. Abnormal due to LBBB.*

C: Why not LV hypertrophy? He has LAD, ST-T changes, possible LAA, and nearly voltage criteria. But with LBBB, we are not able to make that diagnosis. The conduction abnormality itself may cause these changes. The clinical issue is whether the patient has hypertensive heart disease. LBBB generally occurs in a setting of organic heart disease, and there is a history of hypertension. Hypertensive heart disease is likely, and an echocardiogram would sort it out.

Questions and Answers

1. A 72-year-old man comes to the emergency room with severe chest pain that began abruptly 2 hours ago. It was as severe at its onset as it is now and is described as sharp and stabbing. It is anterior in location, without radiation, and there is no change in it with inspiration or movement. There is a long history of poorly controlled hypertension. On examination, he is diaphoretic and obviously uncomfortable. Blood pressure is 140/90, and pulse is 104 beats/min. Pulses are equal in both arms. The chest is clear, and he has a soft diastolic murmur. The electrocardiogram (ECG) shows ST segment elevation in inferior leads (similar to practice ECG A15). Chest x-ray shows clear lung fields and possible widening of the mediastinum. All blood work is pending.

   All of the following should be done quickly, *except*
   A. Intravenous recombinant tissue plasminogen activator therapy.
   B. Beta-blocker treatment to control blood pressure and tachycardia.
   C. Morphine therapy.
   D. Intravenous nitrate therapy to lower blood pressure.
   E. Transesophageal echocardiogram.

2. A 68-year-old man who had MI 6 months ago complains of increasing fatigue, mild dyspnea, and "feeling bad" for 2 weeks. An echo after MI showed ejection fraction 30% and anterior hypokinesis. There has been no recurrence of chest pain. Current medicines include a beta-blocker, angiotensin-converting enzyme (ACE) inhibitor, furosemide, aspirin, and simvastatin. On examination the pulse is about 120 beats/min and grossly irregular, and blood pressure is 114/70. There is no jugular venous distention, but there is abnormal hepatojugular reflux. There are rales at both bases, and on cardiac examination he has no murmur or gallop. The ECG shows anterior Q waves and new atrial fibrillation. What is the best management at this time?

303

A. Increase the furosemide dose and check electrolytes in 1 week.
B. Add digoxin and check the level in 1 week.
C. Add warfarin and follow International Normalized Ratios.
D. Start warfarin, digoxin, and flecainide.
E. Admit to hospital for intravenous diuresis and anticoagulation.

3. Which of the following therapies for hyperlipidemia work by increasing the number of hepatocyte low-density-lipoprotein (LDL) receptors?

A. Low cholesterol diet
B. Cholestyramine
C. Simvastatin
D. All of the above
E. None of the above

4. You are seeing a patient with aortic stenosis. Which of the following would favor medical therapy rather than surgical correction?

A. LV ejection fraction = 26%.
B. The patient is 78 years old.
C. The patient has no complaints and describes no change in exercise tolerance.
D. A and C
E. A, B, and C

5. A 59-year-old woman with lung cancer and metastases to bone and liver is evaluated for lightheadedness. She is cachectic and tachypneic. Heart rate is 130 beats/min, and the ECG shows sinus tachycardia. Blood pressure is 95/40. You notice that her pulse volume varies with the respiratory cycle (it seems to decrease with inspiration). There is marked jugular venous distention, lungs are clear, and there are no murmurs or gallops. There is no peripheral edema. Chest x-ray shows clear lung fields and mild cardiomegaly. Which of the following will improve her symptoms?

A. Direct current cardioversion
B. Intravenous furosemide
C. Intravenous morphine
D. Intravenous heparin
E. Pericardiocentesis

6. A 62-year-old woman had anterior MI treated with angioplasty yesterday; she was in pulmonary edema at the time of treatment. You are called to the intensive care unit to evaluate hypotension. There has been no recurrence of chest pain, and the ECG is unchanged. The resting heart rate is 110 beats/min, and blood pressure is 75/40. A pulmonary artery catheter is in place, and you get the following measurements:

Right atrial pressure, 14 mm Hg
Pulmonary artery pressure, 45/25
Pulmonary capillary wedge pressure, 25 mm Hg
Cardiac output, low

Which of the following is the best therapy for her hypotension?

A. Normal saline, 200-mL bolus
B. Salt-poor albumin
C. Isoproterenol
D. Dopamine
E. Phenylepherine

7. Which of the following therapies has *not* been shown to improve survival in selected patients with coronary artery disease?

A. Aspirin
B. Simvastatin with target LDL < 100 mg/dL
C. ACE inhibitors
D. Sublingual or oral nitrate therapy
E. Beta-blockers

8. Which of the following therapies has *not* been found to help patients with diastolic heart failure?

A. Digoxin
B. Preventing tachycardia
C. Controlling blood pressure
D. Relieving ischemia
E. Cardioversion for atrial fibrillation

9. An important issue when evaluating new congestive heart failure is distinguishing ischemic from nonischemic cardiomyopathy. Which of the following may help sort this out?

A. History
B. An S_4 gallop on physical examination
C. ECG
D. Echocardiogram
E. All of the above
F. None of the above; a perfusion scan or coronary angiogram is needed.

10. The following therapies for heart failure caused by dilated cardiomyopathy may relieve congestive symptoms. Which work by raising cardiac output?

A. Digoxin
B. Nitrates
C. ACE inhibitors
D. Diuretics
E. All of the above
F. A and C

1. **Answer: A**

   The patient is having inferior myocardial infarction (MI), but other features of his illness place dissection of the aorta high among differential diagnoses. The character of pain is typical. An absence of pulse deficit in the arms and no radiation of pain to the back suggest that the dissection is limited to the proximal aorta. A murmur of aortic regurgitation is common with proximal dissection. The intimal flap probably has occluded the right coronary artery, causing infarction (anterior MI is rare with dissection). Thrombolytic therapy could lead to disaster. Beta blockade, pain control, and nitrates constitute medical therapy for acute dissection, and they are useful for myocardial infarction as well. If transesophageal echo is not available, either computed tomography or magnetic resonance imaging would work.

2. **Answer: E**

   New-onset atrial fibrillation is responsible for decompensation in this patient with borderline heart failure. Low ejection fraction increases the risk of stroke with atrial fibrillation, and there is a strong indication for warfarin therapy. Because of his rales and elevated heart rate, hospital admission is warranted (you could argue for outpatient therapy for a patient who is more stable). Flecainide and other class IC antiarrhythmics are contraindicated by the low ejection fraction; the best antiarrhythmic agent would be amiodarone (which is less proarrhythmic in patients with left ventricular [LV] depression). Cardioversion will be needed, as loss of atrial kick has precipitated his heart failure. That should be delayed until he has had 6 weeks of anticoagulation.

3. **Answer: D**

   With each therapy, there is a drop in the amount of cholesterol available to the hepatocyte. The liver cell responds by pulling more cholesterol from the circulation, and this is accomplished by "upregulating" the number of LDL receptors. Resins like cholestyramine bind cholesterol-rich bile salts in the gut, blocking their enterohepatic circulation. The net effect is a deficiency of cholesterol in the hepatocyte.

4. **Answer: C**

   In general, it is safe to delay therapy for aortic stenosis until a patient becomes symptomatic. Low ejection fraction does not contraindicate surgery; repair of aortic stenosis is the ultimate afterload reduction therapy, and ejection fraction can be expected to increase after surgery. Low ejection fraction would be an argument for surgery. Advanced age is not a contraindication to valve surgery; "physiologic age" is more important.

5. Answer: E

She has acute pericardial tamponade, and the pulse changes with respiration indicate accentuated pulsus paradoxus (which should be documented with blood pressure readings). You may not see marked widening of the cardiac shadow on chest x-ray when fluid has accumulated rapidly; the pericardium has not had time to stretch, and tamponade thus develops with a small amount of fluid. Direct current cardioversion is not indicated for sinus tachycardia (treat the underlying cause, instead). She has nothing to indicate congestive heart failure. Pulmonary embolus can present with lightheadedness, but the clinical setting and pulse findings point to malignant pericardial effusion and tamponade.

6. Answer: D

The patient has cardiogenic shock. Her LV diastolic pressure (the wedge pressure) is already high, and volume expanders (saline or albumin) will precipitate pulmonary edema. Phenylephrine, an α-adrenergic agent, is a pure vasoconstrictor; she is already vasoconstricted. Isoproterenol is a vasodilator and may aggravate hypotension. Dopamine or dobutamine are catecholamines that stimulate contractility and raise cardiac output, the best of these choices. Another possibility is the intraaortic balloon pump, although this has not been shown to improve survival. Even with ideal medical therapy, her mortality risk is high.

7. Answer: D

Nitroglycerin has not been found to improve survival or prevent MI. ACE inhibitors prolong survival for those with ischemic cardiomyopathy, beta-blockers improve survival after MI, and aspirin and aggressive LDL lowering are effective for all patients with coronary artery disease.

8. Answer: A

Most patients with diastolic dysfunction have LV hypertrophy, and many of them have hyperdynamic contractility. Inotropic therapy (digoxin) makes it worse. With tachycardia, diastolic time falls, reducing the time for ventricular filling (I suppose an argument could be made for digoxin to control the ventricular rate with atrial fibrillation). Hypertension and active ischemia both increase diastolic stiffness. The stiff ventricle is especially dependent on atrial contraction for filling; with atrial fibrillation cardiac output may fall 30% or more.

9. Answer: E

A history of heart attack and Q waves on the ECG suggest ischemic disease as the etiology of heart failure. Patients with dilated cardiomyopathy have S_3 gallops; an S_4 gallop indicating a stiff ventricle is consistent with ischemic heart disease (as well as hypertensive heart disease). Regional wall motion changes on an echocardiogram indicate prior infarction, whereas global hypokinesis suggests a nonischemic etiology. I usually have a good idea of what is going on before nuclear or angiographic study is done (for confirmation).

10. Answer: F

Nitrates and diuretics are preload reducers. They lower venous return and thus reduce stroke volume (the patient comes down on the same LV function curve; see Chapter 1). Relief of congestion thus comes at the expense of lower cardiac output. Increasing contractility and reducing afterload both increase cardiac output, raising renal blood flow and allowing spontaneous diuresis. It is interesting that digitalis was initially thought to be a diuretic, as it relieved "dropsy" (severe peripheral edema).

Index

Note: Page numbers with an *f* indicate figures; those with a *t* indicate tables; those with a *b* indicate boxes.

complications of, 58t
diagnosis of, 56–57
endocarditis and, 74
pathophysiology of, 57
treatment of, 57–58
Mobitz heart block, 239–241, 240f
Moricizine
  for MI, 183
  safety of, 233t
Morphine, for MI, 148–150
MR. *See* Mitral regurgitation.
MS. *See* Mitral stenosis.
MUGA scan. *See* Radionuclide angiography.
Mumps, CHF and, 2t
Murmurs. *See* Heart murmur(s).
Musset's sign, 65
MVP. *See* Mitral valve prolapse.
Myocardial infarction (MI), 133–203
  ACE inhibitors for, 151t, 152t, 180–181
  age factor in, 161
  angina and, 121, 185–186, 193t, 195
  angiography after, 170–171, 196–197
  angioplasty for, 171
  anterior, 143f, 143–144
  anticoagulants for, 153–155, 154t
  antiplatelet therapy for, 169
  antithrombotic therapy for, 169
  arrhythmias after, 182–185, 183t, 194t
  aspirin and, 137, 148, 149f, 152t, 154t, 169
  atherosclerosis after, 197
  beta-blockers and, 137–138, 150t, 152t, 184, 232
  calcium channel blockers for, 155, 170
  cardiac enzymes in, 139–141, 140t, 170
  cardiogenic shock after, 171–176, 173t
    management of, 174–176
  CHF after, 2t, 178–182, 180f, 193t
  clinical presentation of, 137–139
  complications of, 171–192, 193t
  conduction abnormalities with, 145–147, 146f
  disability evaluation after, 134, 202–203

Dressler's syndrome after, 139, 187–188
driving after, 203
ECG patterns of, 136f, 141–147, 142f–146f
embolization after, 188–189, 193t
exercise after, 197–202, 198f
exercise test after, 196
exercise therapy after, 197–201, 198f
"false," 147
heart block after, 238f
hemodynamic monitoring for, 155
imaging studies for, 196
incidence of, 133, 137
incomplete, 196–197
inferior, 144
injury from, 134
Killip classification of, 138, 139t, 159t
laboratory tests for, 139–141, 140t
lateral, 145
left ventricular free wall rupture after, 191–192, 193t
left ventricular thrombus after, 188–189, 193t
lidocaine for, 153
mitral regurgitation after, 49, 190–191
morphine for, 148–150
mortality with, 133, 134
new murmur after, 189–192
nitroglycerin for, 150–151, 152t
from noncardiac surgery, 256f, 257t
non-Q wave, 135t, 135–137, 136f
  calcium channel blockers for, 155
  ECG for, 135t, 142f
oxygen for, 148
pain control for, 148–150
pathophysiology of, 133–134
pericarditis after, 186–188
physical examination for, 138–139, 139t
platelet function and, 133–134
Prinzmetal's variant angina and, 126
prognosis for, 134, 170
prophylaxis after, 193t, 197
pseudoaneurysm after, 192
pulmonary embolus after, 189

QRS complex
in heart block, 244f
heart block and, 241, 242f
in nodal rhythm, 218f
premature, 212f
in supraventricular tachycardia, 215–217, 216f
of ventricular ectopics, 229, 230t
QT interval, prolonged, 234–236, 236t
proarrhythmia without, 237
Quincke's pulse, 65
Quinidine
safety of, 233t
syncope from, 234–236, 236t
Q waves
MI and, 136f, 143f, 155
surgical risks with, 257t
thrombolysis and, 162

Radionuclide angiography (RNA), 12b, 24
for angina, 109–110
for left ventricular dysfunction, 35
Rales
CHF with, 18–20, 19f
crackles vs., 18
MI and, 138, 139t, 159t
Ramipril, 151t
Raynaud's phenomenon, 123
Recombinant tissue plasminogen activator (rt-PA), 168. See also Plasminogen.
heparin after, 169
indications for, 168–169
Reductase inhibitor, 116t
Regurgitation. See specific valves, e.g., Tricuspid regurgitation.
Reiter's syndrome, 2t
Reperfusion. See also Thrombolysis.
arrhythmias with, 157
assessment of, 170
injury from, 157
pathophysiology of, 156–158
reocclusion after, 157–158
risks with, 159t
Reteplase, 168. See also Recombinant tissue plasminogen activator.
Retinopathy, thrombolysis and, 165
Revascularization therapy, 120–121, 123

Rheumatic heart disease (RHD), 2t
aortic regurgitation with, 63
mitral stenosis with, 43
stroke risk with, 222
Rheumatoid arthritis, 2t
Right ventricular dysplasia, 234t
Right ventricular hypertrophy
diagnosis of, 267t
ECG of, 268f
Right ventricular infarct syndrome, 144, 159t, 176–178
cardiogenic shock with, 173t
clinical course of, 178
diagnosis of, 177
pathophysiology of, 176–177
treatment of, 177–178
Romano-Ward syndrome, 236t
Roth spots, 71
rt-PA (recombinant tissue plasminogen activator), 168–169

SAECG (signal averaged ECG), 194t, 195
SAM (systolic anterior motion), 66, 68
Sarcoidosis, 2t
SCD. See Sudden cardiac death.
Sclerosis, 2t
Septum
ablation of, 68–69
hypertrophy of, 68t
interventricular, 5
Sestamibi, 109b
Sexual activity, after MI, 201–202
Shock. See Cardiogenic shock.
Sick sinus syndrome, 245
sinus bradycardia with, 209
Signal averaged ECG (SAECG), 194t, 195
Simvastatin, 85t
Sinus bradycardia, 209–210
Sinus tachycardia, 209
MI with, 185
Sleep apnea
CHF and, 2t
sinus bradycardia with, 209
Slow ventricular tachycardia, 228t, 229
Smoking
atherosclerotic risk from, 81–82, 82t
cessation program for, 84t
Prinzmetal's variant angina and, 123